Introduction to The Technique

A Holistic Guide to Wellness for Chronic Pain

By:

Juliet Cameron

Table of Contents

FOREWARD

Chronic pain affects over 50 million people a year, or 1.5 billion people worldwide. Any way you look at it that's a lot of people suffering. The cost of treatments span over 100 million dollars per year. You could say that we are a nation with a serious affliction. Most of us are aiming for a cure like a shot in the dark. After enduring doctors, physical therapy and pain medications we are often no better off than when we started. Short term effects may be present but in time our pain increases and so does the medication.

Suffering with chronic pain is no joke. It can stop your life. It disrupts everything from sleep to physical mobility and inherently produces a low quality of life. Ninety percent of all people over the age of forty will be diagnosed with some form of chronic pain. It seems downright unfair that in the second part of our life when we are ready to go out and enjoy the fruits of our labor we're bench bound. Most people accept this as a normal phase of life but the truth is we are meant to remain in an optimal state well into our years. So what happened?

The world we lived in changed and as a result, so did the people. We have become a condition of commercialism and it's produced disastrous consequences. Quick, processed foods have become the standards in a high stressed environment, subjected by teaming violence and pollution. We are now a product of this rat race where healthy living is a bargaining ideal.

Decades of undoing have taken us out of the organic garden and humanitarian farms and into an addictive, low quality of foods. As a result, sickness and disease are dramatically on the rise with no sign of recovery *unless* we be become aware of its intention. It seems that it's not enough to know that healthy eating is good for you. If that were the case, billions of dollars in processed food industries would cease to exist. So I've taken a different approach.

I believe that knowledge is power. Now you can take what is given to you and make your own choices. I cannot make anyone become a healthier, happier, more vital individual, despite my best efforts. But, I can give you what works and what has been proven successful many times over. The rest remains with you. I can assure you however that continuing on the path of habitual behaviors will consistently produce a decline, either rapid or steady, in your longevity and your overall quality of life. This his book was written to stop the cyclic insanity that causes millions of people to suffer every day from unnecessary disease and consequence.

We as a nation have been lied to and I will be hushed no longer. There is little to no profit in a vital, happy world of fit thriving people. Our current circumstantial design is no accident. The very foods that have been commonly placed upon your table making proclamations of being good for you, are made for one purpose only, to keep you sick and addicted. Unless you have plucked your own pesticide free vegetables and fruits from your garden or hail them from a local organic farmer/ store you are at the mercy of toxicity. The same goes for any meats consumed from commercial farms. This may sound extreme to you and that's okay, but I challenge you to acquire the knowledge and after doing so, make your own assessment.

Before we go any further, I would like to share how I came about to this place where I was no longer willing to accept the corruption of society. Sometimes it takes coming to the end of your road before things become clear. This is how it happened for me.

PART ONE

The Road to Recovery

In my early twenties I began to notice changes. I was exhausted and struggling to keep my weight down. I was consumed with trying anything and everything. I tried the grapefruit diet, the cabbage diet, the no sugar diet, the vegetarian way, you name it I did it. And I was incredibly frustrated. Despite that I'd been a dancer and an avid exerciser for the past ten years, nothing had changed. My body was angry, inflamed and in constant pain. Sound familiar?

I saw just about every medical doctor I could think of and wasted $8,000 to hear the same old spiel, "We don't know why this is happening but take this medication and see if this clears up. I'll see you back in a few weeks."

I was put on an anti-depressant to help with pain and prescription strength anti-inflammatories. I was given labels for my illnesses, Fibromyalgia, Irritable Bowel Syndrome, Interstitial Cystitis, Hashimoto's Thyroiditis, Osteo-Arthritis and Pre-Menopause before the age of thirty. I was in so much pain that I took to getting around with a cane. How did this happen? I had worked so hard to eat right and exercise.

I can say that at this point I became temporarily insane. Being so frustrated with my body and hearing the doctors recite the same things despite my condition I became enraged. For all the swelling and extra weight I was encouraged to work out harder and diet more. I was down to eating two small meals a day and drinking up to a gallon of water. Oh, and I should mention that my workouts were exceeding far what is healthy for the most fit individual.

Here was a typical day's schedule. I got up and ate a piece of fruit and chased it with three big glasses of water. I then worked out as vigorously as I could for a least an hour and a half. I got a shower, at a salad and drank more water. I then set out to do my second part of exercise which was dance for another hour. I drank more water and then did thirty minutes of yoga. I was completely exhausted but instead of resting, I drank coffee to keep me going. I then ate a light dinner and did my last thirty minutes of working out before I took a shower and went to bed. On a typical day, I worked out anywhere from three to five hours. When I mentioned this to my doctors they looked at me like I was lying and gave me a skeptical smile. Keep at it, they said, and start walking.

To no avail, I continued to get worse and in 1998 I became deathly ill and took to my bed. I will say that what one experiences during this stage of life is downright intense. I experienced things that would otherwise be considered crazy by anyone who wasn't open to receive the possibility of our immortal essence. I questioned everything and in the end, I felt terribly alone.

Even with my partner who worked meticulously around the clock to accumulate enough money needed for a necessary surgery to save my life, nothing could've prepared me for the visions and the very real words that came from my doctor. "I'm only giving you three days. We have to operate now."

I was fortunate enough to make it in time but what I hadn't counted on was the aftermath. Detox was equivalent to insanity. I had grown tired of listening to the traditional, medical doctors and stretched my approach I wanted to get well and it was going to take making a change.

My story really begins here. After being told by doctors there was nothing more they could do for me, I was placed on a heavy detox by a holistic physician. What I was left with was a crippled body. I was told to accept this and to reach out to others who were in similar distress so that I could better cope with this reality. I wasn't buying it.

I sat down on my living room floor amongst a layer of yoga mats. Even with the carpet beneath me, my body was too tender to sit without lots of cushioning. I tried all of the modern methods of exercise which seemed to cause more pain and inflammation. What was I doing wrong? I'd been teaching aerobics for years and was professional dancer. Now, I was an absolute mess.

I began to list every type of exercise regime and configuration possible. I had nothing else but time and my drive was simple. I wouldn't stop until I found what healed me. There was no failure. I could only go up from here. I pulled from aerobics, Pilates, Yoga, muscular training, general flexibility and dance. I drew out patterns and charts of what hurt and what challenged me. After a few days it hit me. I'd been focusing so intently on the exercises and the need to succeed that I wasn't *really* listening to what my body needed.

I needed to ask myself some valid questions. Where did I hurt the most? What places were locked and stiff the second I got out of bed and what pains shook me awake from an already interrupted sleep? What were the connections to movement, stress, and mental attitude? It was all important.

I began to understand. There were areas that held onto pain and literally refused to allow the rest of the body to get relief until they were *unlocked*. These muscle groups didn't just respond to any kind of exercise either. Movements had to be sympathetic.

I spent months going back and forth documenting what worked and what didn't. I'd been on a roll and then wham, I'd add something that caused pain and inflammation and I'd have to start all over from the top. It was maddening. I learned a whole new level of patience, I tell you.

It took months of a torrent of emotions from screaming, to crying to cursing but I realized that the tension I'd been holding was now released. It had been part of it. I measured success by the grace and forgiveness of the mind into the physiology of the body. They were connected. I also took notice to tempo in movement from one pose to the next. It turns out that slow and easy is the key. As the body healed, progressions were possible and finally, The Technique was born.

After two weeks, I began to notice a rapid improvement. I was stoked. There was not a thing in this world that could've stood in my way. I no longer needed the cane and returned it to its rightful owner. The swelling was leaving and so was the pain. I felt a strange charge, an energy I hadn't felt present before. I was getting stronger. You better believe there was no stopping me now.

In two months, my overall stamina, grace, strength and flexibility had exceeded beyond what I had experienced in my early twenties. Was this for real? I had to keep going and really put it to the test.

In three months I was crazed with a surge of strength and energy. I was back on the big stage performing again. I had proved the doctors wrong! I will tell you this. Dancing is my passion and it's the one thing that ignites my soul more than anything else, so being able to do it again was absolute bliss.

I was hired to perform for Anne Rice at her Vampire Ball in New Orleans. No one could've believed that I was completely disabled only three months ago, nor could they ever comprehend the joy and gratitude I experienced. One thing was for certain. By the end of the show, after receiving a standing ovation, I knew that I had to give this to others. Happiness is never really appreciated until you are able to share it.

As a wellness teacher, I've made it my passion to incorporate The Technique into each of my classes. I have been privileged to work with so many who care about their health and wellbeing. And since I am only one person, I decided it was high time to write this book so that I could get this information out to the masses. No one should live in pain, feeling like there is no hope.

The information provided here is part of an integral system and it's designed to heal and open the body right away. The physical portion is brief and very simple. It should be practiced daily. I have reserved other postures for guided class respectfully, since everyone is different and chronic pain is a case sensitive issue. I need to see you in order to help you on your path to physical recovery. Safety is my most important concern and so the postures I've given you are the easiest to execute without my fearing that may do them incorrectly. Let's get started.

Nutritional Health

All pain and disease comes from an imbalance in the body and almost all of these disruptions occur from an inability to properly assimilate vital nutrients. There have been countless reports and evidence supporting real miracles with a change in eating habits. I neglect to use the term diet since such a word holds negative and restrictive connotations. But, what happens when think you're eating right and you're still sick? That a clear indication that something is still amiss. When we are digesting, assimilating and absorbing essential nutrients, our body heals and does so rapidly.

The human body is designed to function its most optimum level. It will do anything and everything to heal regardless of the abuse we put it through. For example, a smoker will awaken with a smoker's cough. That's because during the hours of sleeping the body gets the message that poisons are not present and makes a rapid push to expel toxic mucus from the lungs. Once the person lights up, the body slows the process signaling that it is once again under attack.

Now this happens with everything. Diets high in sugar change the PH levels making the body more acidic. This is just one of the breeding grounds for producing cancer, the other being high levels of resentment and stress. This is no secret. Cancer patients undergoing treatment are heavily discouraged from ingesting sugar of any kind with the exception of minimal amounts of fresh fruit juices extracted from a juicer. We will get more into the benefits of juicing later.

Cancerous bodies have been ravaged and intensive therapy must be insured to drastically change the balance to become alkaline. A more alkaline body equals a healthy body. But here's the scary part, sugar is put into almost every process food imaginable. You will be hard pressed to avoid it. That brings us to one of our nation's biggest culprits.

High Fructose Corn Syrup

High fructose corn syrup, also known as HFCS was first developed in the 1970's. Constructed in a laboratory, it's much cheaper to manufacture and is highly addictive, giving big business a huge profitable margin. This process is done through method known as chemical enzymatic engineering and don't be fooled, there is nothing natural about this substance.

According to Dr. Bruce Ames, one of the most prominent nutritional scientists in the world, HFCS can trigger a wide range of inflammation and obesity. It is one of the substances in fact fed to lab rats to fatten them quickly so as to study obesity related illnesses.

Refined cane sugar and HFCS are lethal when consumed in large doses. What considered a large dose? Well, it's small than you think. Our ancestors consumed no more than 20 to 30 grams of natural fruit and vegetable based sugars in a **year**. The body understands the organic matrix of these foods and can break them down efficiently, utilizing it for resourceful energy. Today we quite a different story.

Our nation consumes on average 70 to 80 grams of refined sugar in a **day**, with an alarming rate of 120 to 150 grams ingested by our youth. There is no way our body can hand that kind of overload and not become ill from it. With high fructose corn syrup prompting massive cravings, our brains have no idea they're being sabotaged by something as equally enslaving as cocaine and heroin. That is no exaggeration. These artificial sugars change the chemical signals in the brain, creating an immediate feel good response. That's why people continuously consume them in elevations of larger doses. This is how the business was designed. It's cheap to make, can be mass produced in large quantities and is highly addictive which is perfect for repeat business. Unfortunately, your ill health as a result was not part of the concern.

High fructose corn syrup was also constructed so that the body cannot properly digest it. In fact, it goes straight into the blood stream and is taken into the liver. This causes a huge surge in insulin which is the hormone responsible for fat storage. Repeated spikes like this inevitably cause type two diabetes.

Other terrifying factors include little tidbits like these. High fructose corn syrup has been known to puncture the intestinal lining, causing toxic bacteria and undigested, putrefied foods to leak into the bloodstream. This results in an instant inflammatory reaction, opening the doorway for diabetes, cancer, cardiovascular disease, obesity, liver damage, dementia and rapid acceleration of aging in the body. And, if that's not enough, consider this. HFCS contains 50% of mercury, a deadly poison causing permanent damage to the brain and nervous system. How many pregnant women and children are ingesting this without knowing the consequence?

My strong advice to you is to avoid this stuff like the plague. Nothing is worth the disasters this unfood creates. And personally speaking, I'm not into gratifying big business with the sickness of our nation just so they can become wealthy. It's time to get back to healthy, conscience living.

To sweeten our foods, let's use what our bodies can read and digest. Savor honey, *real* maple syrup, stevia and fresh squeezed fruit juices. Retrain the palate to light up to the rich flavors of living wholesome foods, those foods that make us shine from the inside out.

We do our best eating foods in their most natural state. It also pays immeasurably to eat seasonably. We are programed as each species with an internal radar and our bodies adjust accordingly. Our bodies will naturally hunger for what's adaptable for certain climates during certain times of the year. To do anything else, throws us off. So wait until the summer time to eat that watermelon and focus on foods that grow during natural harvest.

Milk Does a Body Good or Does It?

Milk contains lactose which is a sugar disaccharide, composed of glucose and galactose. Lactose is found in **all** dairy foods and is definitely known to suppress the immune system damaging our "T helper" cells. Significant studies have deduced that lactose is linked to Osteoporosis, heart disease, obesity, cancer, allergies and diabetes. It's interesting to think about as doctors still insist that dairy products are still the best way to get calcium. Not true. Milk drinkers and diary consumers have some of the weakest bones on the planet with vegetarians surprisingly having the strongest. Hum, there must be something to that.

The only species that benefits from cow's milk is a baby calf. Seems reasonable, right? This is because milk is structurally made for bovine offspring that weigh up to ninety pounds at birth and grow to a staggering thousand pounds by adulthood. We are nowhere close to this formulation. Human beings are born into this world much smaller and variably reach no more than 200 lbs. during maturity.

By comparison, cow's milk and human milk are predominately different. Human milk contains a rather low protein count for easy digestion but is rich in necessary amino acids and is also constantly changing according to baby's needs. The entire composition of human milk was created for optimal needs up until the age of three years.

After this age, we no longer require the enzyme to break down milk sugar or milk protein because of weaning. Now we can obtain our nutrients from solid food sources. Digestible calcium, vital minerals and vitamins are present in green leafy vegetables, root vegetables, fresh fruits, nuts and seeds. Flesh should be consumed sparingly from a humane source and should always be organic and hormone free.

Diary has been responsible for more allergies imaginable and it strikes me as odd that allergists don't advocate a diary free health plan to their patients. But then business would be..... (You fill in the blank). Here's a list of illness caused by dairy products.

Illnesses caused by milk:

> * **Hay Fever**
> * **Asthma**
> * **Bronchitis**
> * **Sinusitis**
> * **Arthritis**
> * **Type 1 Diabetes**
> * **Intestinal Distress**
> * **Infertility**
> * **Leukemia**
> * **Autism**

The effects of lactose are well known and any doctor who doesn't bring these to the table cares little for the patient.

Cow's milk contains casein which is a thick, gooey and course protein found in milk. It creates a mucous slime in the gut, causing severe inflammation. This substance is actually used to make the most industrious glue in the world. It's no wonder our bodies can't possibly handle the burden of ingesting this without consequence.

In addition it's important to note that cows release toxins through their milk. As a result cows are treated with these hormone cocktails:

> **Pituitary**
> **Hypothalamic**
> **Steroid**
> **Thyroid**

They are also given Gastrointestinal Peptides, rBGH (Recombinant Bovine Growth Hormone) which is linked to human breast cancer, colon and prostate cancer.

Pus is also found in milk. National averages equal at least 322 million cell counts per glass. As repulsive as this is to think about it's necessary knowledge. This grotesque substance is linked to partuberculosis bacteria, known to cause Crohn's Disease.

Blood cells are also found in cow's milk. Up to 1.5 million white blood cells per milliliter are permitted as acceptable by the USDA. Due to the cow's constant state of severe stress and sickness, antibiotics are commonly administered. Thirty eight percent of milk is polluted with sulfa drugs but a study from the FDA concluded that fifty percent actually contains pharmaceutical drugs. Is this what we really want in our bodies?

Let's get well by eating well. Here are some great alternatives to cow's milk.

Rice Milk
Coconut Milk
Almond Milk
Raw Goat Milk
Hemp Milk

*Remember to check your labels. Some products are sneaky and contain high fructose corn syrup.

Artificial Sweeteners

Will the culprits please stand.

Saccharin
Neotame
Acesulfame Potassium
Aspartame
Sucralose

Here's the skinny. When obesity began rearing its ugly head, industries took notice. A great new discovery was plastered all over the media proclaiming that sugar makes you fat. There is truth in that as we discussed earlier but the game was on and new horizon of zero calorie chemicals promised to cure your sweet tooth without gaining a pound.

The nation was splattered with pictures of gorgeous creatures who could enjoy their sodas and candies guilt free, taunting a slim waist line and a socially awesome lifestyle. Funny, those that do indulge encounter the opposite and they wonder why. Isn't the media right? And all too quickly we rest the blame upon ourselves instead of questioning the industries motives.

The body can only process that which it naturally recognizes. The rest attaches itself to fat cells or remains stored in fatty tissue. The fact that our bodies don't really understand how to break it down is no help to us either. This is why it's imperative not to ingest those things made in a laboratory. It's so much harder to get that gunk out of our body let alone dealing with some of these other maladies.

* **Migraine Headaches**
* **Brain Tumors**
* **Mental Retardation**
* **Birth Defects**
* **Epilepsy**
* **Parkinson's Disease**
* **Fibromyalgia**
* **Lymphoma**
* **Leukemia**
* **Memory Loss**
* **Brain Lesions**
* **Peripheral Nerve Damage**
* **Cancer**

Life is challenging enough without adding the potential for any of these. Don't be fooled. Leave the stuff alone.

Gluten

Gluten intolerance affects more than half the nation though I'm willing to bet those numbers are higher. Why? Most people have intolerances and just don't know what to look for. Before I get into the mechanics per say of what gluten does to the body I would like to share with you a few of these heavy hitters.

Gluten is responsible for causing these maladies and as you can see from many of them, they are autoimmune related.

* **Arthritis**
* **Lupus**
* **Cancer**
* **Adrenal Exhaustion**
* **Migraines**
* **Autism**
* **Osteoporosis**
* **Schizophrenia**
* **Dandruff**
* **Psoriasis**
* **Lactose Intolerance**
* **Weight Gain/ Unresponsive to Exercise**
* **Infertility**
* **Manic Depression**
* **Lowered Immune Response**
* **Depression**
* **Dizziness**
* **Multiple Sclerosis**
* **Epilepsy**
* **Neurological Disease**
* **Sinusitis**
* **Yeast Infections**
* **Ringing in the Ears**
* **Body Chills/ Flu like Symptoms**
* **Light Sensitivity**
* **Noise Sensitivity**
* **Insomnia**
* **Massive Fatigue (CFS)**
* **Allergies**
* **Soreness and Body Ache**
* **Inflammation**
* **Celiac Disease**
* **Crohn's Disease**
* **Acid Reflux**
* **Irritable Bowel Syndrome/ Disease**

Gluten destroys the body through way of the intestinal tract. It does so by means of abrasion, erosion and inflammation. Inside the gut live tiny projections called villi which protrude from a protective layer called the epithelial lining. These tiny protrusions are vital for absorbing nutrients and giving us maximum health.

To better understand this concept, let's think of these villi as a sectioned stem. Each part carries with it a unique and important responsibility. The very tip of the villi are always the first to be affected. It produces the enzyme that breaks down lactase. First symptoms of this destruction include a runny or stuffy nose and accumulated mucous in the lungs and throat. Asthmatic problems may become prevalent.

Next down the villi, comes sucrose production. This is responsible for breaking down your sugars. Diseases such as diabetes and hypoglycemia manifest at this level. It's estimated that 25.8 million people suffer from diabetes in the United States alone and that could be turned around with a proper change in diet.

The next part of the villi is responsible for nutrient absorption. When this is damaged, the intestinal wall thins, forms cracks and deteriorates. Toxins then flood the blood stream and poison the system. An increase in acne is usually present. Others usually develop dandruff and psoriasis at this stage.

PH levels cause the body to become acidic, raising the risk for cancer. With the blood and organs now under attack, autoimmune disease is imminent. The intestines are inflamed and swell with fluid. This leads to the appearance of the pot belly or beer gut. Irritable bowel syndrome or disease follow and energy levels plummet. This opens the door to Celiac Disease. Once thought to be purely hereditary by doctors, it's now recognized that this is not always the case.

Fortunately, many companies are rising to the request of gluten free foods and are delivering some very tasty pastas, breads and treats. We've spoken and they've heard. There is one thing you should know and I tell this to all of my students. Expect to crave what's been ailing you. Gluten has a terrible addictive quality but once you realize what's happening, you can overcome it. The cravings don't last once the body starts healing and I promise you, you will begin to feel a lot better.

Check labels and be prepared to be shocked. Gluten is found in everything from soups to barbecue sauce. One of the healthiest things you can do is begin to invest in fresh produce and make many of your meals right from home. Put fresh soups in a crock pot or buy gluten free rice pastas.

Rapid healing comes from eating a variety of fresh wholesome vegetables and fruits as well as organic proteins. In fact our diet *must* consist of up to 70% of high water content veggies and fruits for us to be healthy. Anything less is suicide. I know that might sound extreme but it's true. Our bodies were never designed to live off of lifeless foods that have been processed or biochemically altered in a laboratory.

Eat low glycemic fruits to satisfy your sweet tooth and of course drink plenty of water. Cut out all processed food and leave soda alone. If you have to indulge do so very rarely but honestly opting for herbal teas or fresh squeezed juice is always better.

When you feel you've been left with nothing, it's time to step forward and make a change.

FOOD COMBINING

So all we have to do is eat healthy and exercise, right? Emphatically speaking, this isn't the case. The human body is designed for simple, optimal digestion. Our ancient heritage understood these principles as hunter-gatherers. We chose foods in season and ate for longevity, selecting whole clean foods. To do otherwise would have been suicide in an age when you were either hunter or hunted.

Over time we got lost in a more sedentary world where those of the upper class ate to savor their palates in a variety of culinary fascinations. What began an expression of wealth and diversity led to indigestion, headaches, fatigue and an onset of diseases that sprang rapidly.

We never knew. As doctors scrambled to whip up their potions for symptomatic maladies, humanity continued to eat to its demise. Except....for those still remaining in their indigenous cultures.

It took us centuries to understand the miracles of digestion and it wasn't until the late 1800's that we came around full circle to the principles once considered primitive, redirecting ourselves back to health. Going strong, health and wellness projected an ingenious standard and we began to see a rise in vital wellbeing unseen for decades. That was before the large food industries got greedy.

I could be a quiet mouse and sit on the fence post, not speaking of such things but that won't do anyone any good. The truth is we are the unhealthiest nation in the world and that's depressing, considering America sets their standards in competition with the very best. In truth, we are failing miserably in long term health and winning in obesity, crime, cancer and addictions. Thank God we aren't above changing it.

I have always believed that most of what we need to make an honorable commitment is intelligence and that requires information. Some will continue on their downward spiral to doom but I am certain that is not you, since you are reading this book right now. What brought you to this point is as important as what you do from here. I want you to feel better, look better, think better and have the best quality of life imaginable but it will take dedication from you, for you and no one else.

We have been conditioned for far too long to shorten our life span and line the pockets of big corporate industries. There is power in taking back one's control and declaring your strength as a right human on this planet. So, I won't blow smoke up your butt. It's going to be a challenge, as change usually is. But, the end result is worth its weight in gold. This I promise you.

Nations are plagued with lies concerning disease and illness. We see more time and money spent on laboratory tests that are clearly not working. In fact, the rate of cancer has not changed for the better. Those that are making progress are shushed under the carpet as new age thinkers that couldn't possibly have any footing on reality. After all, they are med school traditionalist. They are naturalist and preventative health care physicians. How could they know anything?

Alternative practiioners stretch to change and that's exactly what it's going to take to bring insight to those once *incurable* diseases. What we are seeing are miracles in doctors who have cared enough and expanded enough to leave the realm of persistent views and have reached to examine what has worked in the past and making amazing adjustments in their skills as holistic providers. I am speaking here about souls such as Dr. Max Gerson who in the late 1800's was looking for a way to heal his ailing migraines and in the process turned the world upside down with his naturopathic findings for curing cancer and disease.

Incredible achievers have saved lives and spawned movements that continue to better the lives of humanity. Jay Kordich is another example. After suffering with a serious illness at the young age of twenty five, took juicing therapy from Dr. Max Gerson which incidentally not only saved his life, but excelled it upon its years. We know Jay most commonly as the Juice Man.

Herbert Shelton regarded taking an approach with the combinations of foods that we eat as matter of honest, digestive reactions. He studied in depth works by gastrointernist and chemists abroad finding hard pressed evidence to sickness and related disease caused by poisoning of digestive organs. Not that this was new information.

For centuries holistic practioners treated the digestive system first in treating and curing diseases. Once the greed of pharmaceutical companies took charge, it no longer became profitable for people to get well. Miserable people are in constant need and that's no accident. All medications that serve to harm keep the ball rolling in the wrong direction. While companies succeed at large, family and loved ones are dying off leaving us with broken hearts and more questions.

What I've strived to do here is take the very best of all that we know on a global scale. There is a common voice and a direct connection to our organic nature and the blessings that were placed upon this earth for us to heal. We are much less likely to *ever* encounter disease in a well body. Does that mean it could never happen? No. We are complex creatures and emotions and lifestyles do play a part as much as the nutritional aspect.

Louise Hay has done beautiful and remarkable work on ascertaining the connection between emotions and the body's physiology. She herself suffered from a terminal case of cancer and beat it just like Jay the Juice Man. The world is full of real miracles and there is no reason you shouldn't be one of them.

You can expect to experience an interesting mix of feelings once you begin this process. Your body will detox very quickly if given the right tools and you should be prepared for feelings of upset and fatigue. Your mind is going to question everything because that's what it does. It's also responsible for addictions, so please understand this. Your first job is to be informed and then to relay this message to your brain that you are doing this for the gold, not for a short term quick fix.

Your mind will tell taunt you with foods that will harm you, delivering messages any way it can to break you. You are going to have to be strong. The good news is that once the detox begins, within a few days, the mind begins to clear itself and begins to quiet. Our mind doesn't comprehend the big picture until we present it and though this might sound strange it is true.

All addictions, habitual behaviors and violence come from the mind, not the heart or the spirit of the soul. It is conditioning, repetitive self-talk and blind action that keep us enslaved. Your mind will clear and it will begin to understand as soon as it's given the signal that things are getting better within the organism as a whole. Be gentle. Don't find anger with the mind. Be like a loving parent who is consistent in doing the best out of love and respect.

Your first week may be tiresome. Don't fret. Take good care as this is a sign of detox. Embrace what's coming in rapid acceleration of energy, strength, endurance, stamina, mental clarity, glowing skin and a radiant life force. That's why you're doing this. You need to be free of pain and affliction. It's no longer a want but a desire that must be attained because you've had enough and it's high time for change.

So, let's get started. Food combining is an essential component to health. Did you know that our bodies produce more than one type of stomach acid to digest food? The acids needed to digest proteins are far different from those needed to break down carbohydrates. If two incompatible foods are taken in at the same time then one of those foods will be delivered into the intestines partially digested where fermentation and purification results.

The decaying byproducts irritate the bowels from excessive overgrowth of bacteria producing the breakdown of proteins into amino acids. The amino acids are then destroyed and what's left are a host of poisons such as indol, skatol, phenol, phenylpropionic and phenylacetic acids, fatty acids, carbon dioxide, hydrogen, marsh gas, hydrogen sulphide to name a few. Most of these are exported from the body through the feces while the rest is left to leave by way of the urinary tract and sweat glands. This is how foul smelling stools and bad body odor occur. It is our bodies design to purge impurities from us any way possible.

Inflammation in the intestinal lining occurs as a result and damages the gastrointestinal tract. Most people experience stomach upset, gas, heartburn and acid reflux and unfortunately we have been convinced that this is not a big deal. But what's being experienced is the effect of disrupted chemical processes in the stomach and gut. Fatigue, irritable bowels, stomach disorders and the like are a result of that. Ignoring it or masking the symptoms with drugs only further the damage and what ensues are intestinal cracks and holes in the lining which leak toxic poisons into our bloodstream. This is how most doctors keep you coming back and this is how you end up on the surgeon's table or with severe gastrointestinal diseases.

I often hear people refute gastro related illnesses to foods but this only happens because they can't foresee themselves living happily without certain foods. As long as we continue to believe that eating incorrectly will suffer us no consequence, we are doomed to become ill and feeble in the wisest of our years.

If we look at people across the globe and study those that live strong and healthy well into their hundreds, we see that their diet is clean. They grow and ingest a predominate variety of fresh vegetables and fruits. They eat lean meat and fish caught from clean waters or happily grass fed cattle. The second thing you will notice is that they are united in their community and that stress levels are low due to support from family and friends. They acquire enough sleep and work with love and purpose. We will get into this more throughout the chapters but for now I'd like to put a bug in your ear.

The Technique is designed to open you to all of these aspects not just one or another. We are complete beings and must be treated as such. We have talked about the importance of basic nutrition, now let's learn more about the construct of the actual combinations of foods that work together and which ones don't.

To remove all confusion, I'm going to categorize foods into proteins, starches, fats, fruits (sweet, acidic and sub-acidic) and vegetables (both high water content and mildly starchy).

Proteins

Nuts
Dry Peas
All Organic Meats
Dry Beans
Soy Beans
Eggs
Avocado (Is a Complete Easily Digestible Protein)
Nut Butters
Olives
Seeds
Yogurt (Goat)

Starchy Carbohydrates

Dry Beans
Dry Peas
Potatoes (All Kinds)
Hubbard Squash
Banana Squash
Pumpkin
Caladium Root
Jerusalem Artichokes

Mild Starchy Vegetables

Cauliflower
Beets
Rutabaga
Carrots
Salsify

Non-Starchy Vegetables (High Water Content)

Lettuce
Celery
Collard
Spinach
Endive
Chard
Chicory
Okra
Cabbage
Cucumber
Cauliflower
Broccoli
Sorrel
Brussels Sprouts
Asparagus
Dandelion
Egg Plant
Escarole
Summer Squash
Green Beans
Sweet Peppers
Turnips
Tomatoes
Parsley
Cilantro
Water Cress
Zucchini
Bamboo Shoots
Water Chestnuts
Sprouts (Alfalfa and Bean)

Syrups and Sugars

Brown Sugar
Raw Sugar
Maple Sugar
White Sugar (Best to Avoid This)
Cane Syrup
Milk Sugar
Honey

Fats and Oils

Olive Oil
Nut Oils
Soy Oil
Corn Oil
Canola Oil
Vegetable Oil
Sunflower Oil
Tallow
Sesame Oil
Cotton Seed Oil
Butter

*(Stay Away from All Unnatural Butters and Spreads)

Most Nuts (These are a Healthy Source of Fats)
Avocados (High in Omega 3 Fatty Acids and 18 Essential Amino Acids)
Organic Meats

Sweet Fruits

Banana
Persimmon
Dates
Dried Figs
Mangoes
Cherimoya
Raisins
Papaya
Cherries
Thompson and Muscat Grapes
Prune
Sun Dried Pears

Acid Fruits

Orange
Limes
Grapefruit
Sour Apple
Pineapple
Sour Grape
Pomegranate
Sour Peach
Tomato
Sour Plum

Lemons
Blackberries
Raspberries
Strawberries
Tangerines
Tangelos

Sub-Acid Fruits

Fresh Figs
Apples
Pears
Apricots
Sweet Cherries
Huckleberry
Sweet Peach
Sweet Plum
Blueberries
Kiwi
Nectarine

Melons

(Eat Melons Alone)

Watermelon
Pie Melon
Musk Melon
Banana Melon
Honey Dew
Crenshaw Melon
Christmas Melon
Casaba
Persian Melon
Cantaloupe
Nutmeg Melon

Eat high water content vegetables with proteins.

Eat mildly starchy vegetables with proteins.

Eat starchy carbohydrates with fats and oils.

Eat starchy carbohydrates with mildly starchy vegetables.

Eat high water content vegetables with starchy carbohydrates.

Eat high water content vegetables with fats and oils.

What to avoid.

Eat all fruits alone. You may eat sweet fruits with other sweet fruits. The reason for this is simple. Digestion of fruit does not occur in the stomach. It actually takes place in the small intestines. If you eat any other food with fruit, digestion in the small intestines is staled due to the time your stomach needs to digest the other foods. As a consequence the fruit ferments in the gut and creates toxic waste, resulting in inflammation and an increase in yeast overgrowth.

Do not eat protein with fats and oils.

If you drink goat milk or eat yogurt, eat it alone as its protein structure is different from both nut and meat protein. It's best to consume only one kind of condensed protein at a meal.

Do not drink liquid with a meal. It dilutes your digestive juices that start in the mouth, making the breakdown of food less effective. At first you may feel bothered by this but within two days your salivary glands get the message and begin producing a better quality of saliva and signals the stomach to make high quality, digestive acids. Remember to take your time and chew your food well. Certain signals are released from the brain upon swallowing and you don't need your stomach working harder than it has to. Quick digestion delivers immediate transference to energy.

Healing Herbs

Spices have been used since as far back as 50,000 B.C. These vital sources are super rich in phytonutrients. They protect against disease and work wonders for longevity, not to mention they taste great. So lavishly use them in foods or make them into teas. Delicious.

Vanilla: This aromatic, sensuous herb is an anti-carcinogen. It targets and destroys cancer cells and has been found to terminate the advance of broad spectrum human cancers.

Nutmeg: Delivers pain relief, relieves anxiety and lowers high cholesterol.

Black Pepper: A spice addition that aids in digestion, helps prevent and treat cancers and arthritis. It reduces inflammation, stimulates brain function and steadies balance in the elderly. Black pepper has even been attributed to helping overcome the addiction of smoking. It lowers blood pressure and helps prevent heart disease.

Cinnamon: A fantastic anti-inflammatory. It lowers blood sugar for those with Type 2 Diabetes. It reduces high cholesterol, keeps the gums and teeth healthy and happy, improves digestion and alleviates sinus congestion associated with colds and allergies. Cinnamon increases blood circulation, helps prevent bladder infections and is also an aphrodisiac.

Turmeric: A powerful and ancient antioxidant and anti-inflammatory. It can be used as a poultice to reduce swelling on the skin. It heals the liver and aids in the healing process for hepatitis. It also increases bile production in the liver and protects it from toxicity.

Ginger: A spicy, aromatic delectable, ginger improves muscle tone and function in the digestive tract. It also helps in the prevention of nausea and vomiting, which has been used for centuries by women ailing from morning sickness. It relieves diarrhea, stomach aches and gas. It may also help in the prevention of cancer and Alzheimer's.

Basil: A savory herb that tones the cardiovascular system. It's also very beneficial for those suffering from asthma or colds as it stimulates the lungs. Basil calms the nerves, relieves headaches, lowers fevers and heals skin infections.

Oregano: A super anti-fungal, anti-inflammatory, anti-microbial. Not much gets by this baby. Oregano is a dynamic healer. It's used for swollen or sore throats, insomnia, headaches, and intestinal problems. It also destroys intestinal parasites. Oregano contains a powerful 42 anti-oxidants, more than apples, 12 times more than oranges and 4 times more than blueberries. It's also an amazing uterine tonic. For that reason, women who are pregnant should limit their consumption until birth.

Garlic: This pungent herb regulates cholesterol levels, tones the heart and lowers blood pressure. Its anti-bacterial property is used to treat minor infections.

Star Anise: A fragrant stimulate for the senses, Star Anise is used as a digestive aid and an immune booster.

Cardamom: This ancient spice was once used as a natural deodorant. Internally it boosts energy, helps in digestion, opens the lungs and alleviates asthma and bronchitis. It also helps lift a bad mood. Every office space should have one.

Cloves: Mysterious and seductive, clove improves digestion, eases diarrhea and stomach cramps.

Fennel Seeds: Fennel soothes the intestines by encouraging the production of gastric juices. It's a calmative for the nervous system and heals the intestinal muscles.

Cumin: A great immunity booster, Cumin improves liver function which is imperative to a healthy body. It lessens gas and aids in digestion.

* Note that most of these healing herbs naturally care for the entire system with many of them concentrating on healthy liver and digestive function. It would seem that Mother Nature knows her stuff and is consistent in helping the body keeps its integrity.

Juicing

Juicing is a supercharger. There is no faster way to get massive amounts of healthy nutrition in the body in such a short amount of time. Juicing enables us to consume in one glass what it would take us all day to eat. Our biggest problem as a nation is that we are over fed but malnourished. How does this happen?

Consuming empty nutrient foods contain high calories but minute traces of vitamins or minerals. Satisfaction is only temporary as the body's need for vital food is still not met. This creates a pattern of cyclic hunger while gaining weight. Our bodies are starving, relaying a message to our brains that we must be in a time of famine. Thus, pounds are not burned but held onto for the sake of survival.

Now a great many of these lethal foods which we talked about earlier are highly toxic and cannot be digested or delivered throughout the body. Therefore the only way to remove those substances is through detox. To be well we must fuel our bodies with its necessary means and remove the poisons which prohibit proper organ function.

Juicing does both.

From the moment digestion occurs in the mouth, the body immediately sends signals to the body and brain that pure nutrition is being processed. This is why we chew the juice in the mouth a little bit before we swallow it. The receptors are open and the body is charged to accept it. Remember we are designed to heal and yearn for it especially when we are in the throes of illness or disease.

In just fifteen minutes the nutrients are completely digested in the stomach and passed into the intestines where it begins to work its magic. Dispersing into the cells, the body now begins to cleanse, strengthen and detoxify the blood, nerves and organs. This is why some people feel very tired when they first begin to juice. The body literally pools energy to work as efficiently as possible. Detoxing poisons from the body becomes high priority.

For this reason I suggest you make sure that you allow yourself time to adjust for a few days, listening and honoring your body's requests. If you need to rest then do so. Yogic prana breathing should be practiced for a few minutes every day since this is one of the ways to quickly remove toxicity from the body. If you are completely exhausted (and mind you this is temporary) do some light yoga postures to keep the blood circulated and the body oxygenated.

It only takes a few days for the body to awaken and you begin to notice things taste different, smell different and colors are actually more vibrant. It's hard to know just how incredible you feel until you are in an optimal state of health and you experience it for yourself. No matter what I say or how I say it, it's going to be your journey that makes this worth it.

People all across the world are healed by juicing every day. There is no chronic illness or disease that juicing can't improve. Your body hungers for it that much. What we can't do is wait until we're on death bed before we opt for change. That should never be the end factor that changes your mind because then you're toying with a divine miracle that may or may not come for you. We must be proactive *now!*

It's inevitable that disease will inhabit a body uncared for. There is no chance that it will miss you. Any form of chronic illness or disease will manifest and that's not hype it's truth. The body will continue to struggle until it is weakened into an ill state.

The onset may begin with headaches, skin rashes, irritability, foggy thinking or the like. You may even link these things to stress and come to believe that they are temporary, believing there will be relief when you have the right medication or the time to release some stress. This is not right forward thinking. We have to start out with a commitment in the mind to love ourselves enough to do what will give us happiness, vitality and youth. Then we have to put the right things in our bodies to make that happen. Then we need to follow through with mindfulness, learning to surrender to the greatness of ourselves. We do this by letting go of stress as an observer and not one who is swept up in a cycle of pain. It takes practice and what we know from being human is that anything practiced long enough becomes habitual. We might as well make our habits good ones.

Have you ever heard people reminisce about the stories of others who smoked and drank and lived to an old age? In their own defense they reasoned that the individual they knew seemed well enough and happy enough, and if it worked for them then they could do it to. What people may have forgotten is that we filter what we want to see through the eyes of little knowledge. In other words, we cannot step into another person's body and literally experience their day, feeling all of their emotions and physical challenges. We assess what we think we know and then we make a story to fit it.

There is no veracity to smoking, drinking, stress, exhaustion or a sedentary lifestyle bringing great health, wealth and happiness. It's important to ask yourself, what is my definition for happy living? You need to be clear and realistic. External circumstances never equal happiness. Pleasure starts from the inside by the fuel we give it with our thoughts and actions. If we believe for one second that we can shove cheese burgers, fries and shakes in our mouths every night and live without suffering, we are in for the letdown of our life.

Our world is drawn toward beauty, the healthy and strong. Have you ever noticed how people that shine have others flock to them? People throw themselves upon the mercy of those that are thriving. Quite the opposite is true when you are down on your luck or ill. People avoid you and eventually you feel invisible.

It's an interesting phenomena. We gravitate toward those that have what we want and desire. The same thing happens when we feel great. You draw success toward you. I think everyone wants to feel needed and respected. You can hardly do that when you're shuffling about overweight, in pain, bitter, distressed and wheezing. So if you need this vision for transformation, let it help you. If you want to attract light into your life then you can strive to be that which everyone desires which is to be happy and healthy.

If you find yourself struggling then I want you to ask yourself a very important question. Would you risk being miserable in exchange for feeling fantastic? Why not? Now listen to what comes up. That is your drive and that is your focus.

Here are few good things to note on your journey into juicing and healthy eating.

1) Understand that in the early stages your brain may drive you crazy. Remember it's purging. Give it a few days to get a handle on what's happening within the body. To keep the craziness down, limit your television viewing or restrict it until you feel stronger. Junk food commercials are rampant on the tube. If you love entertainment, rent a movie or indulge in music. Surround yourself with supportive friends and family. Once you feel strong and can see things as they really are in a world of commercial push, then you will be less likely to ever return to that way of life.

2) Train yourself to think clear. Get into the habit of shopping in places that promote healthy, organic foods. Venture to local earth and food friendly farm stands when you're hungry. Stock up on living food goodies and savor each bite. Remember to give your taste buds time to change. If you've been eating poorly for a while things may taste bland or strange. It takes a few days for your palate to open and once it does, it's heavenly.

3) If you crave sweets, indulge in a fresh fruit juice. It will satiate your sweet tooth plus boost your body with rich vitamins, minerals and antioxidants. Now that's something no candy bar or scoop of ice cream can give you.

4) Commit to do something active every day. Your body will remove toxins faster and you will be fueled with feel good endorphins.

5) Take time to get proper sleep. Allow yourself time to rest and recover. Studies have shown that sleep actually dissolves stress hormones and deep sleep metabolizes cortisol and epinephrine. Lack of sleep drains the immune system and the adrenals. It also causes intense inflammation in the body which residually leads to weight gain and additional body pain. Sleeping for only three to four hours equals two to three pounds of inflammatory, liquid body weight which will convert to body fat. A twenty to thirty minute cat nap everyday can do wonders for the mind and body.

Here are a few juicing recipes to get you started. Refer to the back of the book for reading suggestions for more great recipes. Please note that some recipes contain a mix of fruit and vegetables. This is because juice is digested quickly in the body and sugars do not have time to ferment in the intestines.

It's important to juice with organic ingredients. Pesticides and herbicides are absorbed very quickly into the bloodstream during juicing so it's best to avoid them.

Apple Pineapple Ginger

1 Organic Apple Sliced and Cored (Apple Seeds are Poisonous)
1 Cup of Fresh Pineapple with the Skin Removed
1/2 Inch of Fresh Ginger

Blueberry Grape

1 Handful of Fresh Seedless Grapes
1 Cup of Fresh Blueberries

Cucumber Celery

4 Medium Carrots with the Greens Removed
1/4 Medium Cucumber with or without the Skin

1 Stalk of Celery
1 Apple Sliced and Cored
1/2 Lemon

Easy Greens

1 Head of Romaine Lettuce
1 Stalk of Celery
5-6 Leaves of Kale (or Spinach, Dandelion or Parsley)
2 Apples Sliced and Cored

Parsley Veggie

1 Cup of Fresh Parsley
1/2 Apple Sliced and Cored
2 Carrots
3 Celery Stalks

Spinach Veggie

1 Cup of Fresh Spinach
1/2 Cucumber with or without the Peel
2 Stalks of Celery
3 Carrots
1/2 Apple Cored and Sliced

Refreshing Greens

1/2 Cucumber with or without the Peel
1/4 Sliced Honeydew Melon with the Rind Removed
1 Handful of Seedless Grapes
1 Large Handful of Fresh Spinach
A small Sprig of Fresh Mint
1/2 Lemon without the Peel

Carrot Kale

6 Carrots
A handful of Fresh Kale Leaves

Our bodies will always let us know when things are out of balance. Here is a chart taken from the works of Dr. Lynn Tan, "You can Regain Youth & Health through Detoxification & Rejuvenation"

Development of Chronic and Degenerative Diseases

Acute Stage of Elimination

Stage One

* Inflammation
* Discharge
* Low Immunity
* Fever
* Colds

Sub-Acute (Poor Health)

Stage Two

* Fatigue
* Stuffy/ Blocked Nose
* Overweight
* Headaches
* Lower Back Pain
* Skin Breakouts/ Blemishes
* Piles
* Constipation
* Digestive Disorders
* Hormonal Imbalances

Chronic

Stage Three

* Migraine
* High Blood Pressure
* Skin Disorders
* Arthritis
* High Cholesterol
* Severe Back Pain
* Ulcers
* Sinusitis
* Asthma
* Weak Sexual Impulses
* Endometriosis
* Infertility
* Tumors/Cysts/Fibroids

Extreme Chemical Deficiency Degeneration

Stage Four

* Heart Disease
* Liver Problems
* Stroke
* Gall Bladder Disease
* Diabetes
* Severe Arthritis & Gout
* Kidney Disease
* Severe Skin Problems
* Lymphatic & Cellular Dysfunction
* Impotence
* Cancer

Little Hidden Secrets in Your Bathroom

Deodorant

When we think of deodorant we search out for the most effective antiperspirant out there. The last thing we want is to be embarrassed by wet underarms or worse, bad body odor. So why do we sweat?

Sweating is a natural, healthy process. It keeps us cool, detoxifies the blood and balances the salts and PH in the body. Under each arm we have lymph nodes which are connected by the lymphatic vessels. Lymph nodes work in conjunction with the immune system and function as filters ridding waste by products from the body. Their roles are very important to vital health. In fact, the action of your lymph nodes can say a lot as swelling can be contributed to signs of fighting off infection or having cancer.

It's incredibly important to allow your body to drain effectively so that toxins are not recirculated by into the bloodstream causing illness. But what does the commercial deodorant do?

All deodorants are designed to dry up perspiration and lock out odor which is novel idea except that the ingredients are precursors to illness and disease. To better understand this formulation and process let's break down the common components in the most typical over the counter product.

Aluminum- Blocks sweat glands. Also known to cause breast cancer and Alzheimer's.

Parabens- Causes breast cancer.

Propylene Glycol- A humectant used for drying out the skin. It was originally created as an antifreeze. It's a neurotoxin known to cause dermatitis, kidney damage and liver damage.

*The National Institute for Occupational Health and Safety warns their workers to avoid skin contact with Propylene Glycol. Warnings include eye irritation, skin irritation with chronic exposure causing gastrointestinal problems, nausea, headache, vomiting and central nervous depression.

TEA and DEA- (Triethanolamine and Diethanolamine) Adjusts the PH levels in the body. It's a carcinogen (cancer causing) and toxic if absorbed over long periods of time, causing liver and kidney damage. It's also known to cause severe allergic reactions and has been banned in Europe.

Triclosan- A skin irritant. Known to cause dermatitis and has been shown to disrupt proper thyroid function and other major hormone systems.

FD&C- Cancer causing carcinogens that cause a multitude of allergic reactions.

Talc- A known carcinogen and linked to Alzheimer's.

There is a safer solution. Many earth, people friendly companies have produced a remarkable variety of natural, nontoxic deodorants. I'm personally found of the Thai natural, unscented deodorant spray. It's very effective in eliminating under arm odor and works even during high excursion. Look into what pleases you but always make sure to check the labels for ingredients. Your under arms are very porous and will absorb whatever you put on them quickly.

The yellow stains that you find on your shirts are actually not caused by underarm bacteria but are a result of aluminum drain. That just goes to show you how much gunk is trying to be excreted from your pits. We don't need our bodies to work any harder than they should have to. Changing to a natural deodorant can do wonders for long term health.

Toothpaste

It's hard to know what to believe when you go to a dentist office and they tell you to pick up the latest tube of commercial toothpaste. After all they use it themselves so how bad could it be? What we've been fed by the media is shocking. The push to deliver cavity fighting whiteners and plaque busting, breath fresheners is everywhere. And we are told time and time again that this is the only way and the best way to keep a happy healthy mouth.

So how do you explain the dozens of indigenous tribes that have the strongest most beautiful teeth in the world? If it's not the toothpaste, what gives them their gorgeous smile? The Wodaabe Tribe and the Masai Tribe of Africa have stunning teeth which are unaffected by age.

Melvin Page D.D.S and Leon Abrams Jr. of *'Your Body is your Best Doctor*,' wrote a compelling 189 page novel depicting the lifestyles of the indigenous peoples in Alaska. Their daily rituals didn't involve actual teeth brushing but only mouth rinsing with pure water. It was noted that as soon as the diets changed from the native standard, adopting that of the western culture, tooth decay became prevalent.

It would appear globally that what keeps a healthy mouth is a healthy diet sustained by the foods eaten in that area. For example, each tribe eats a variety of stable foods that grow well in their climate. They eat no refined sugars or processed foods period. One such tribe may live more solely on fish or fatty meats such as the Inuit while another may consume potatoes, root vegetables and harvested, milled grains. Each food is grown from the earth or caught from the wild.

This being the case, why do dentists and commercials direct to entice us with chemical toothpastes when the number one ingredient, Fluoride, is so dangerous? Fluoride stimulates unnatural bone growth. It causes mutated human cells and stresses the thyroid. It's shown to cause bone cancer and increases the risk of tumors throughout the body. Fluoride both disrupts the function of a healthy immune system and causes Arthritis.

In one family size tube of toothpaste, there is enough Fluoride in it to kill a 25 lb. child. You may also want to read the warning label on the back of the back of the tube. It states: *If accidentally swallowed get medical help or contact a poison control center right away.* The recommended size for use is the size of a pea but how often do you see that accuracy when viewing it on a television commercial?

There are a host of toxic chemicals within a tube of commercial toothpaste and they have been linked to everything from Autism to ADD, Bipolar Disorder, ill health, to mood swings and fatigue. Some chemical components such as PEG - 6, **8**, 12, 32, 75, have been shown to cause developmental and reproductive toxicity, organ system poisoning and endocrine disruption.

It angers me that we are not more informed about what these things do so that we can make an honest decision on whether to use them. So, I'm here to say truthfully, question anything and everything that doesn't come from a natural source and investigate it thoroughly. We are not getting the data we need. It's time to stop this madness. Check your local health food store or go online in search of natural, safe toothpastes. Be careful with some brands as they have been bought out by industrial companies. Whatever you put on your body and in your mouth should not shorten the years of your life or put you're at risk for disease.

Sudsy Sulfates

Last but not least we are covering the ground of both Sodium Lauryl Sulfate (SLS) and Sodium Lareth Sulfate (SLES). Both of these are commonly used in almost every cleaning supply. They're in soaps, shampoos, detergents, toothpastes, hand creams and cosmetics. While these two chemicals act as a foaming agents they hold some pretty heavy consequences.

Sodium Lauryl Sulfate and Sodium Lareth Sulfate are classified as esters of Sulfuric Acid. However, there are at least 150 different names by which it goes under. So recognizing those sulfates can be a bit tricky.

Here are a few different names they can go under.

Sodium Di-ethylene Glycol Lauryl Ester Sulfate
Alkyl Ether Sulfate
Sodium Dodecyl Polyoxyethylene Sulfate
Sodium Lauryl Ethoxysufate
Sodium Polyoxyethylene Lauryl Sulfate
Sodium Dodecyl Sulfate
Lauryl Sulphate Sodium Salt

There has been a great bit of dispute about whether or not SLS or SLES causes cancer. What has been determined is that both of these compounds are commonly contaminated with Dioxane, which is a known carcinogen.

The Journal of American College of Toxicology published a 1983 report stating that concentrations as low as 0.5% SLS or SLES could cause irritation and concentrations of 10-30% caused skin corrosion and severe irritation. It's surprising to note that many of our everyday soaps contain up to 30%, which the ACT report called "*highly irritating and dangerous.*"

Among the most frequent reports to the FDA, shampoos are sited the most. These include incidences of eye irritation, scalp irritation, tangled hair and swelling of the hands, face and arms. Other reports from the AJT state, "*other studies have indicated that SLS enters and maintains residual levels in the heart, the liver, the lungs and the brain from skin contact.*"

Animal studies concluded that only 10% of SLS caused acute corneal damage. According to the American College of Toxicology, "*tests show permanent eye damage in young animals from skin contact in non-eye areas.*" Having said that we should be appalled that most children's shampoos contain levels conducive to adult shampoos even though they promote the "*no tears*" advertisement. We don't even have to get the stuff anywhere near our eyes to be afflicted with permanent eye damage since the maladies are caused from basic skin absorption.

Possible side effects caused by SLS and SLES are:

Skin Irritation/ Skin Corrosion/ Inflammatory Dermatitis
Hormone Imbalance/ Male Infertility
Eye Irritation/ Eye Deformities in Children
Protein Denaturing
Possible Carcinogen

Fortunately, lots of people are taking notice giving rise to products that are both sulfate and paraben free. Search on line or check your local health food store for great alternatives. They will be a bit pricier but remember that SLS and SLES are cheap foamers and that's why the cost of sulfate laden shampoos are low. Paying a bit more can give you more than just a little piece of mind.

PART TWO

PHYSICAL RECOVERY

Level One

Breathing and Awareness

Sit in a comfortable position with your spine tall. Place one hand on your chest and the other over your abdomen. Relax the muscles of the throat. Imagine your throat as hollow bamboo.

Take a clear, full breath through the nose. Allow the air to flow as if pulling through a large straw. Slowly inflate the chest, letting the air fill the abdomen. Feel the lift in the chest and the rise in the abdomen, as if you were inflating a large balloon. Slowly release the abdominals and chest on the exhale. Go at your own pace.

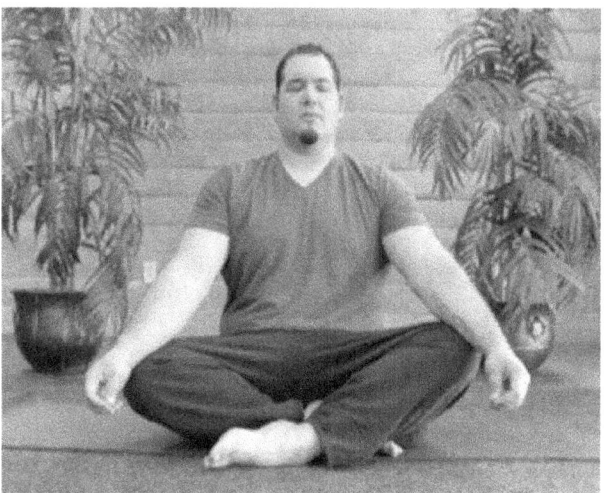

*You may feel a little light headed when you first do this. This is normal. The dizziness is caused by a rapid increase in circulatory oxygen. Take it slow. It will dissipate with time as your body becomes accustomed to higher levels of oxygen.

Do your best to use this breathing in each of the postures. It will fuel the body with oxygen and replenish the cells.

*A note about our model Bryan. After suffering for years with obesity, hypertension, high cholesterol, scoliosis and painful knee and ankle joints, Bryan agreed to do the photos for this book. As these pictures were taken, he'd only been on the program for two weeks and lost ten pounds. His insomnia and depression disappeared. He has once again regained his libido and has a new optimism for life.

SEATED HIP OPENER

Releases Lower Back

Tension in Hip Flexors, Buttocks and Hips

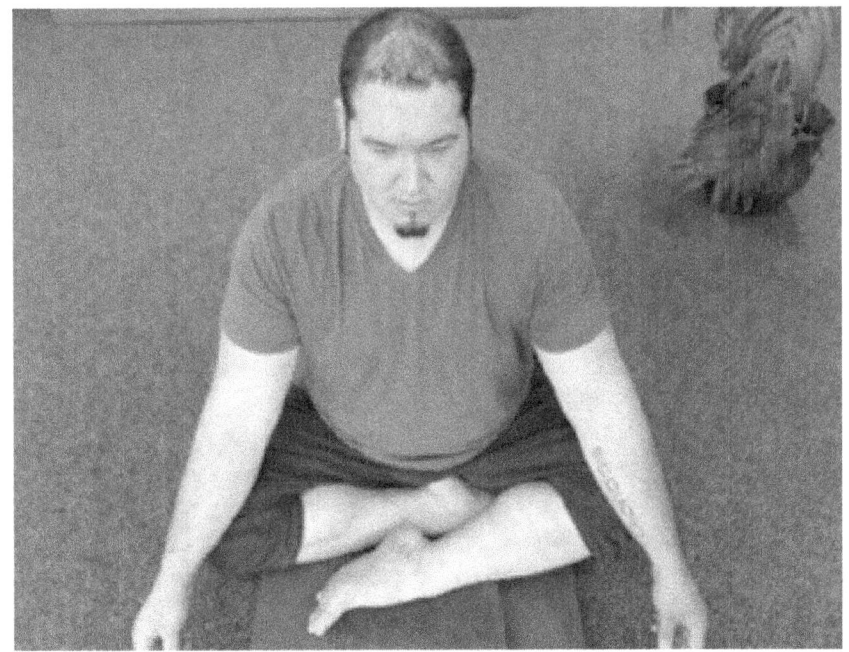

Keep the ankles uncrossed to reduce stress on the feet.

Sit in easy tailored sit with the ankles uncrossed and resting on a folded blanket.

If your hips are tight then your knees may sit high off the floor.

Relax as much as possible and go easy.

Variation with blanket folded under hips and a folded towel under the ankles

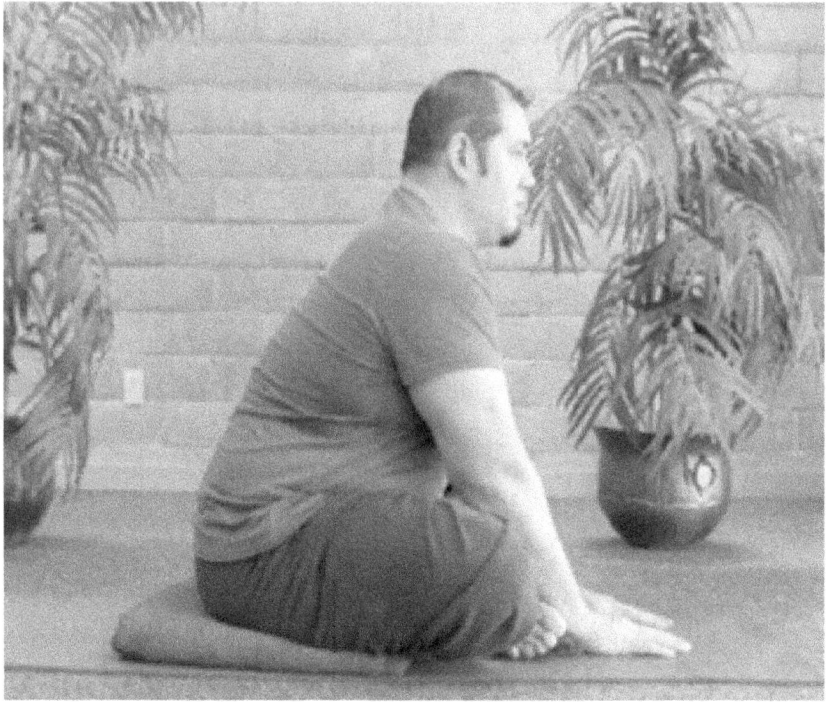

Hinge forward from the hips. The folded blanket beneath the ankles will serve to cushion your ankles. When your hips are tight the ankles and sit bones bare more weight. With time and patience you will open. Breathe clear and deep, relaxing all tension.

Feel the stretch in both hips, opening the entire sacrum. Hold for a count of 15.

*This is usually the hardest time for beginning students.

There's a natural want to be further along than anticipated. However, that's unrealistic. We must all start somewhere. You cannot judge your performance today on what you did in the past.

For example, if you used to be a dancer or athlete and have not been in practice for years; do not expect your body to hold that dexterity. We must work consistently to uphold results.

The good news is that if you were active in the past, your body will remember. With time you may come to once again enjoy some of those things you did in your earlier years.

If you've never been active before, don't fret. Your body has a definite desire to heal and be well. You have just as much chance as anyone else to be free of pain, gain strength and flexibility and to experience a better quality of life.

OPENING THE SIDE GILLS

Lengthens the Erector Spinae

Releases Tension in Lower Back

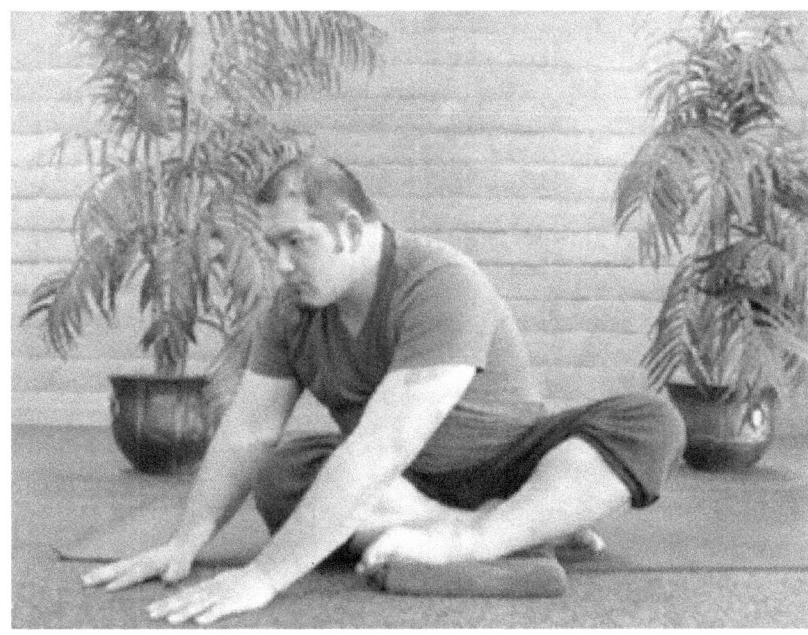

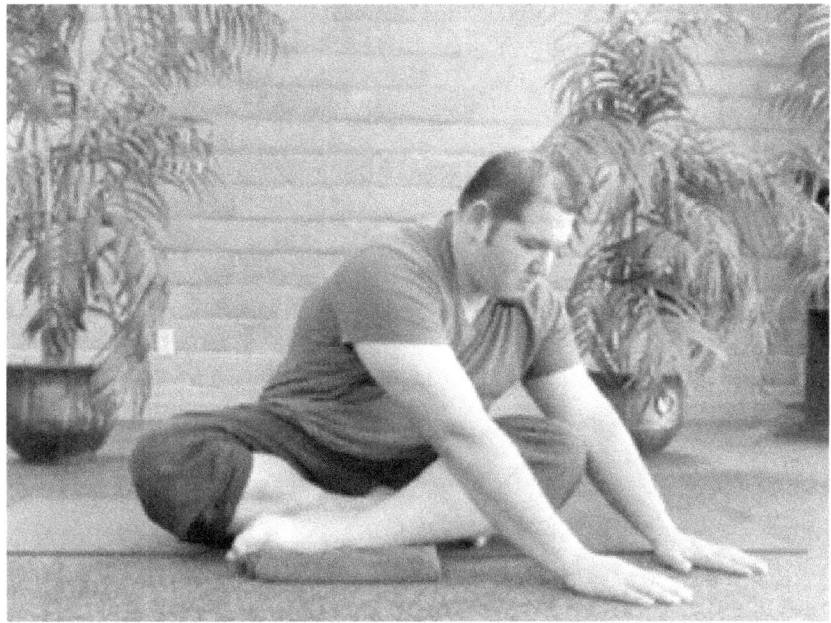

Sitting in easy pose, turn body over the right knee and place palms on the floor. Bend the elbows slightly if able. Feel a lovely stretch all along the left side of the back. Slowly walk through center to the other side and repeat.

Hold each side for a count of 10.

OPEN THE SPINE

Conditions the Entire Spine

Messages Every Muscle in the Back

Front to Back

Rest the hands on the knees.

Start with a straight spine.

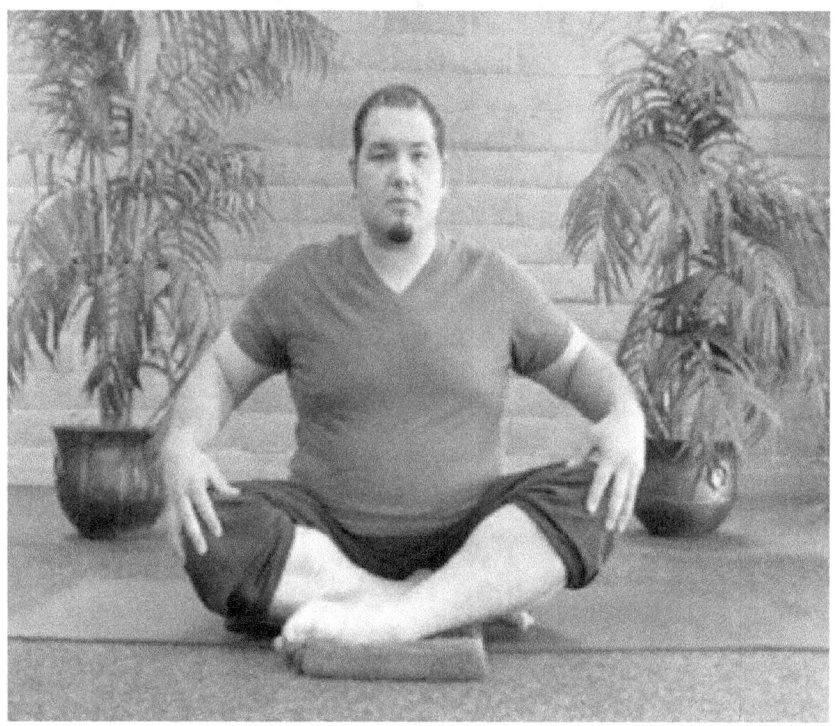

Inhale and press the chest front.

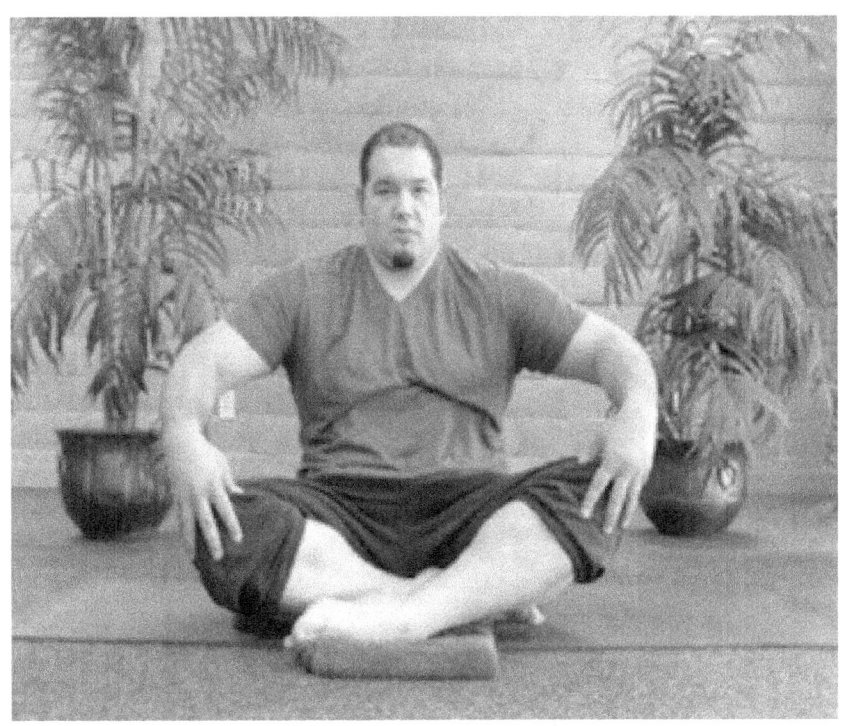

Exhale and press the chest back.

Circles

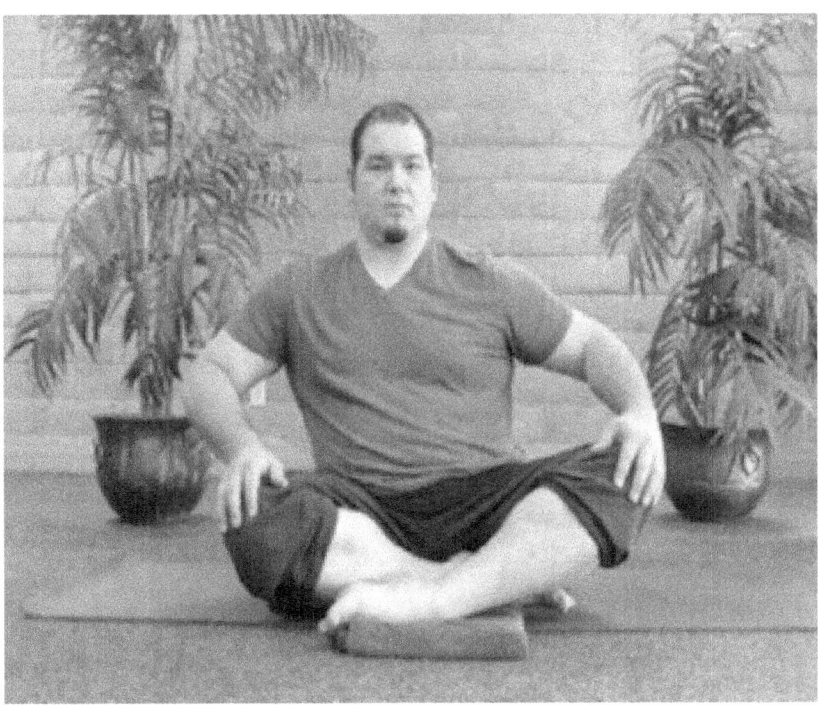

Slide the chest to one side and inhale.

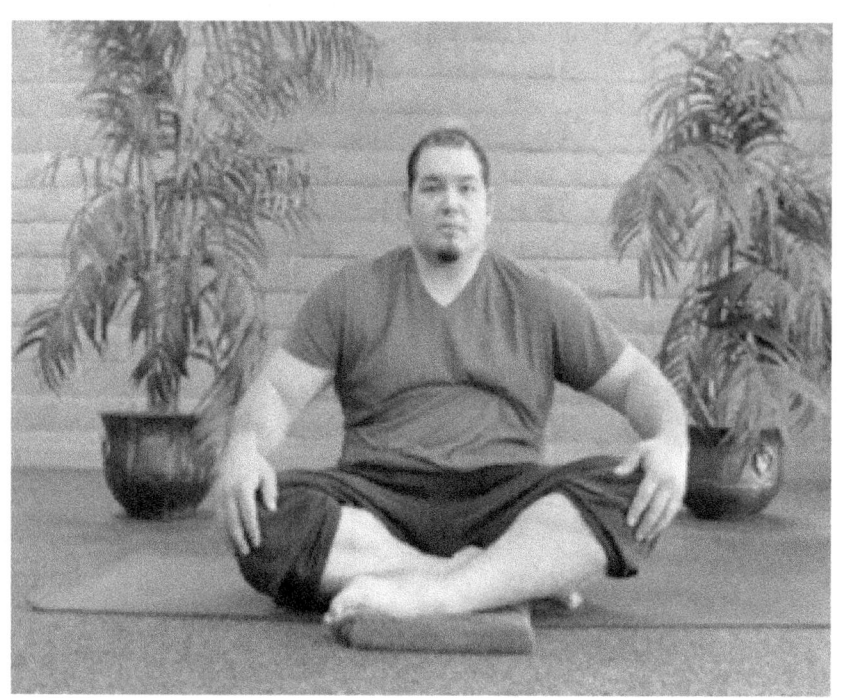

Exhale and press the chest back.

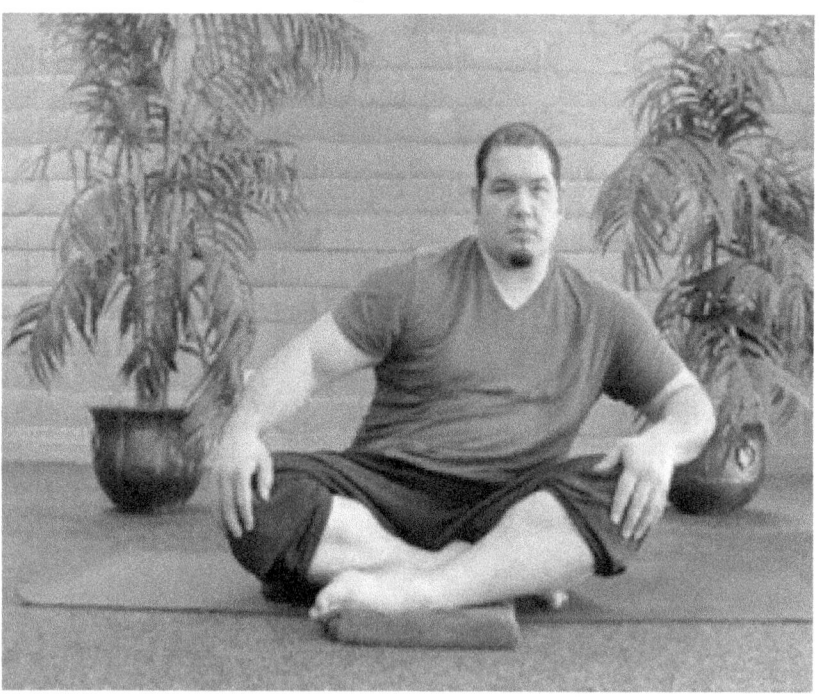

Inhale and slide the chest to the other side.

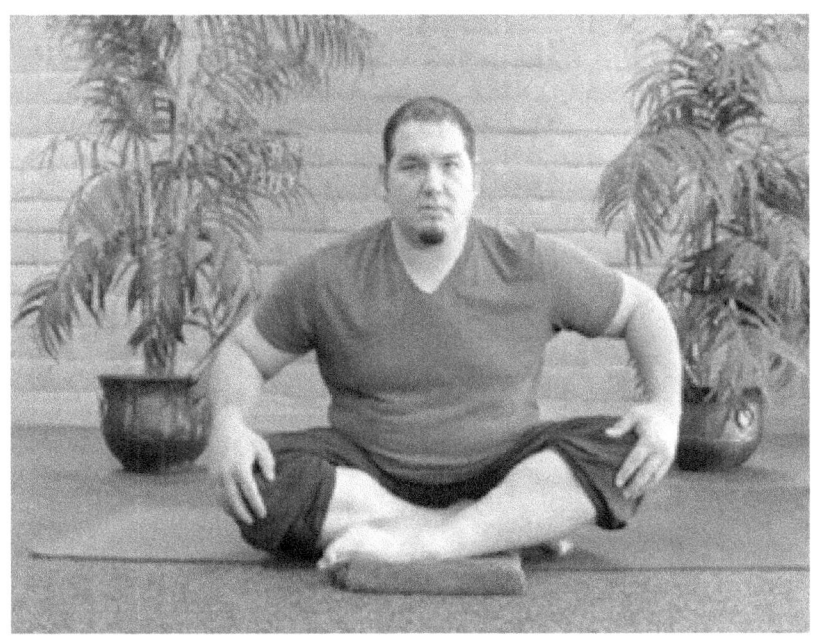

Breathe and stretch the chest front.

Practice your circles 6x.s each way.

EXTENDED SINGLE LEG STRETCH

Lengthens Calf and Hamstring Muscles

Opens the Lower Back

Bend the one foot close to the body and rest it on the inside of the thigh.

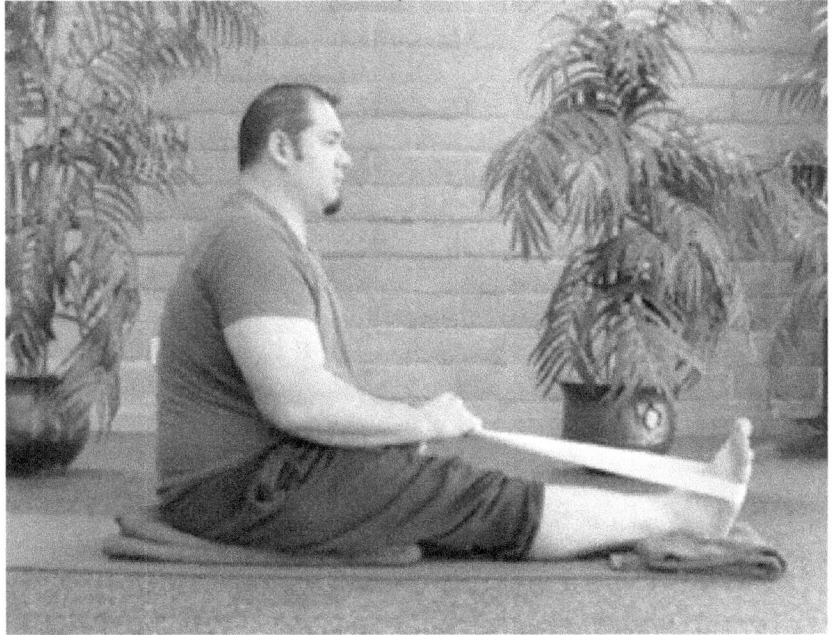

Extend the other leg and wrap either a towel or exercise strap around the sole of the foot.
Keep the spine straight and pull gently on the strap.

Hold for a count of 15.

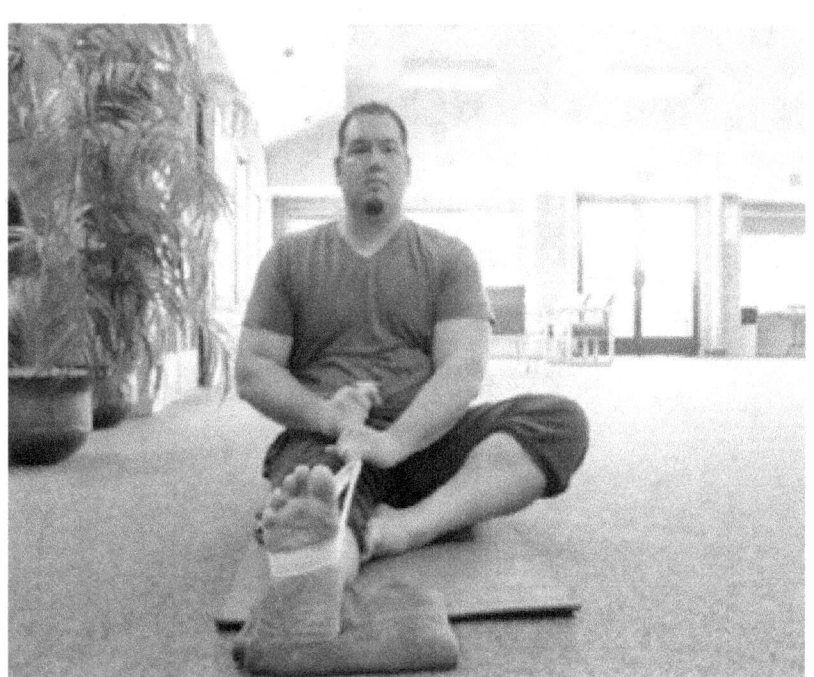

EASY SPINAL TWIST

Opens the Spine

Aids in Healthy Digestion

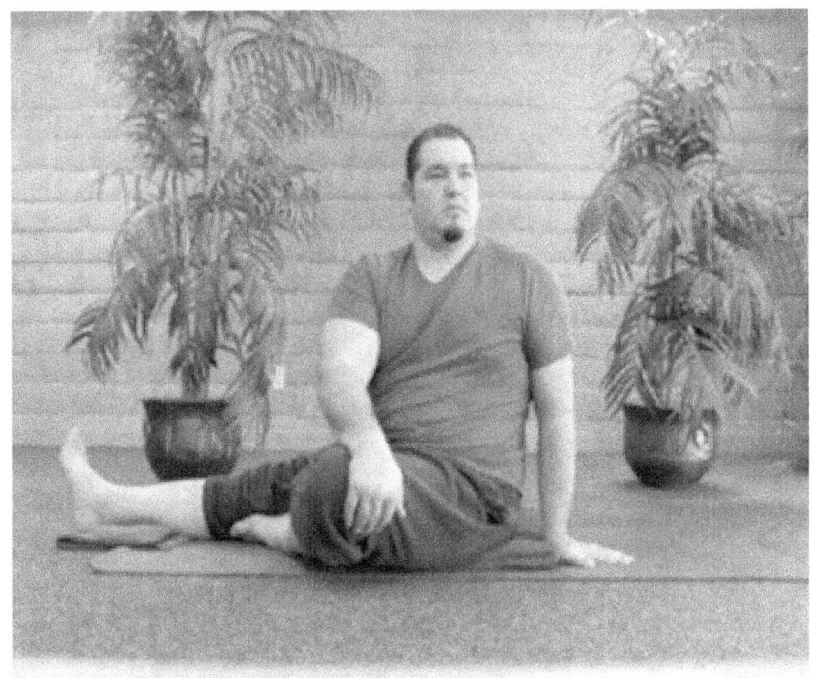

With a straight back take a deep, refreshing inhale. Exhale as you gently twist the body to the right side. The arm behind you stays strong on a lifted hand.

REPEAT ENTIRE SEQUENCE WITH THE RIGHT FOOT IN FRONT

Seated Hip Stretch

Open the Side Gills

Open the Spine Sequence

Extended Leg Stretch

Easy Spinal Twist

<u>OPEN DIAMOND</u>

Releases Hips and Lengthens Adductors

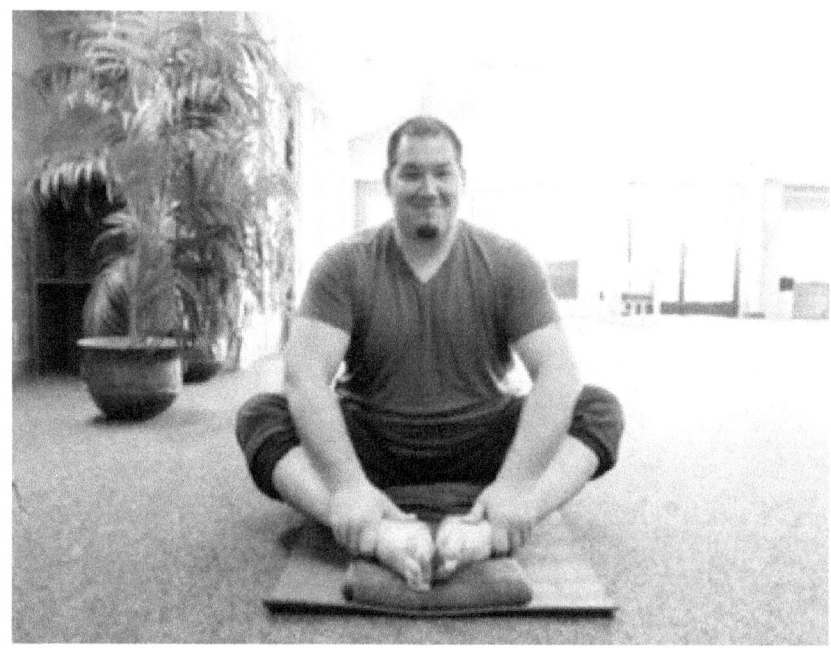

Place the soles of the feet together a few feet from the center line.

Rock side to side and sit tall.

Without collapsing the chest come forward. Hands may rest on the floor or the feet.

Hold for a count of 15

NECK RELEASE

Opens the Entire Region of the Upper Back and Neck

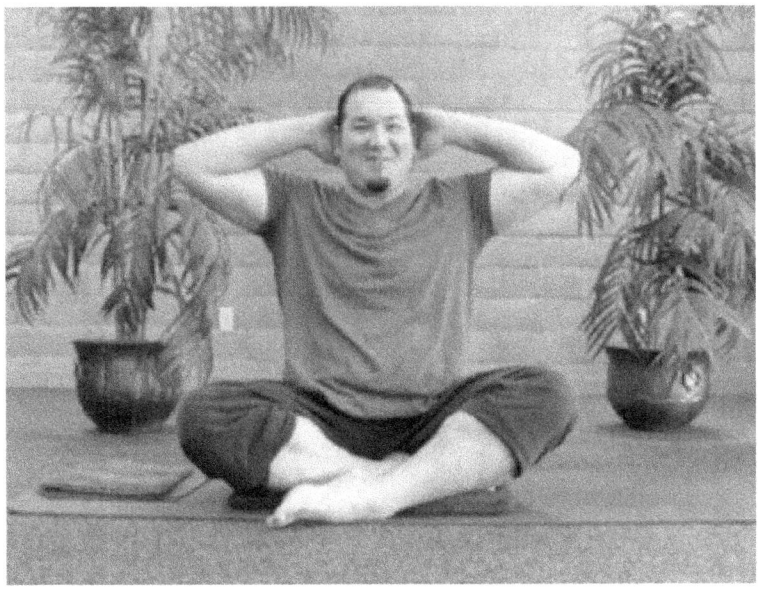

CHIN TO CHEST

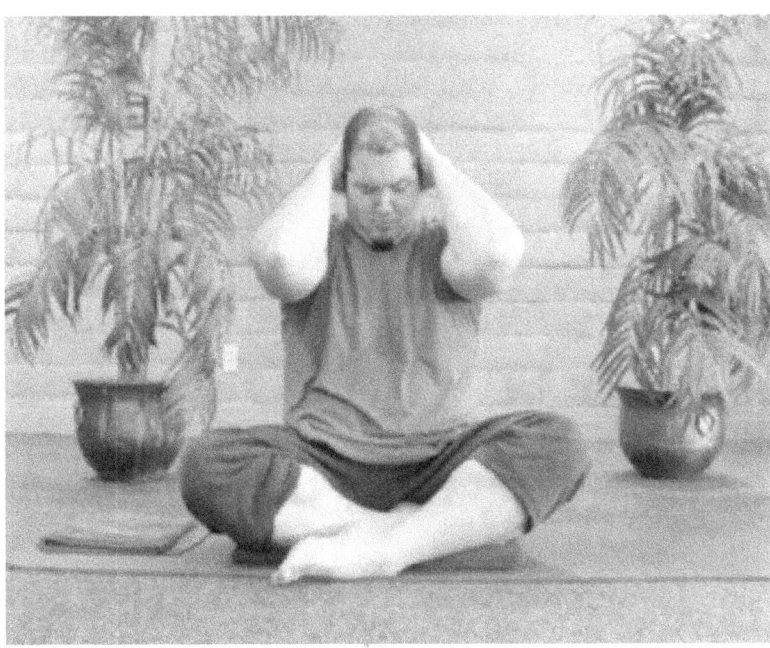

Sit in a comfortable pose.

Interlace fingers behind the head at the base of the skull. Draw the elbows toward each other (they do not have to touch).

Tuck the chin to the chest feeling a deep opening through the neck, upper spine and between the shoulder blades.

Hold for count 10

LIFT AND LOWER

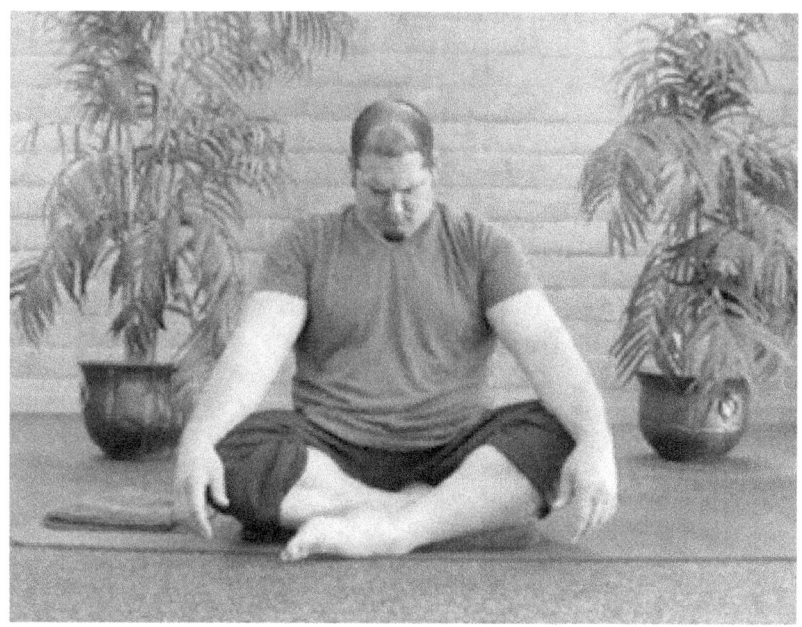

Start with a straight spine exhale and lower the chin to the chest.

Inhale guiding the head upward leading with the chin.

Feel an easy stretch in the throat.

Return to center and repeat.

Repetition of 4

LOOKING OVER THE SHOULDER

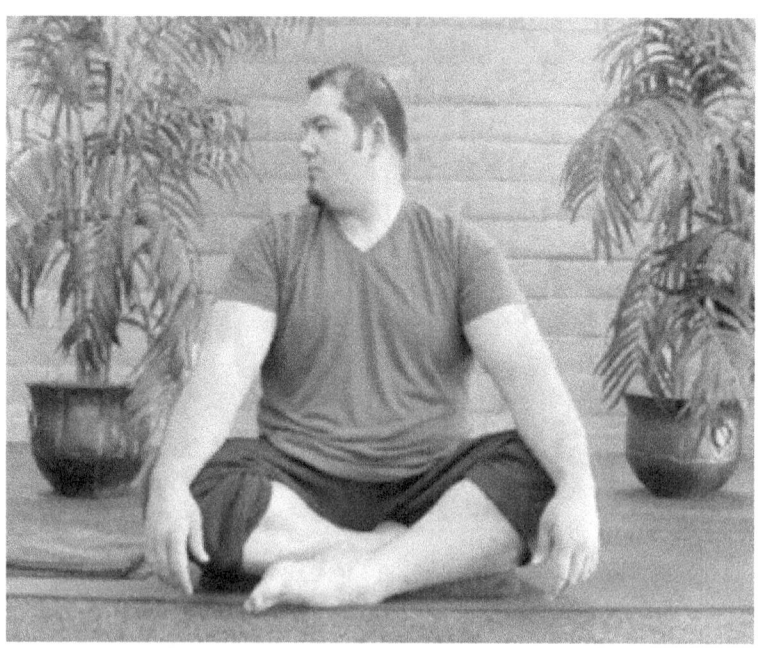

Inhale sitting tall. Exhale and look over one shoulder.
*Do not tilt the head. Keep it level on its axis.

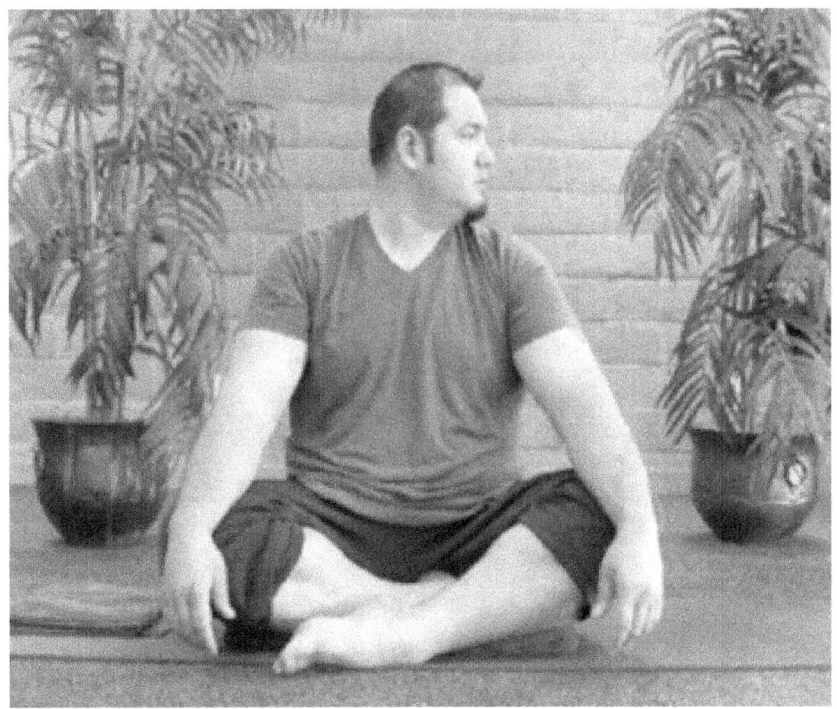

Inhale through center and exhale looking over the other shoulder.

Do repetition of 4

HEAD CIRCLES

Imagine your drawing a circle with the point of reference coming from the crown.

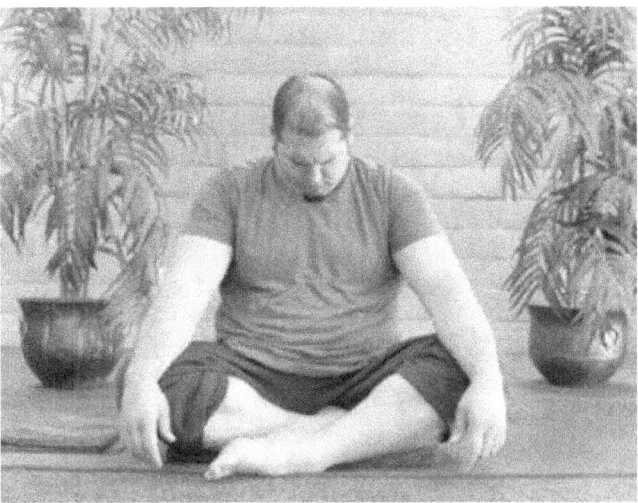

Lower chin to chest and gently guide the right ear to the right shoulder.

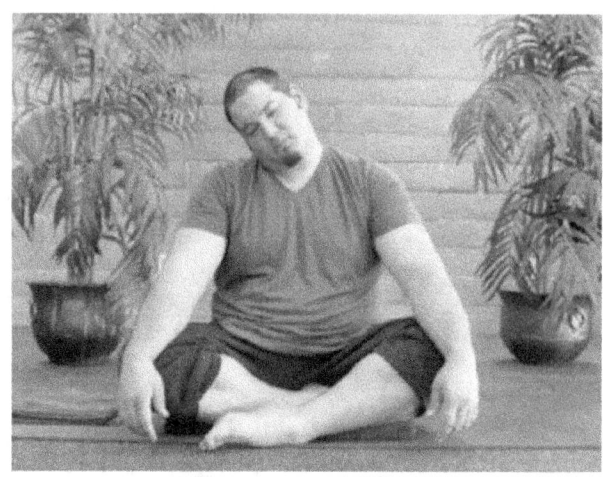

Lean one ear to the shoulder. Remember to breathe.

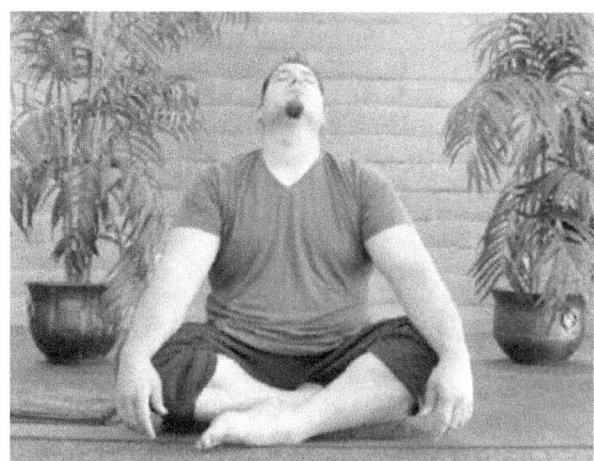

Look up, being mindful not to hyperextend too far back.

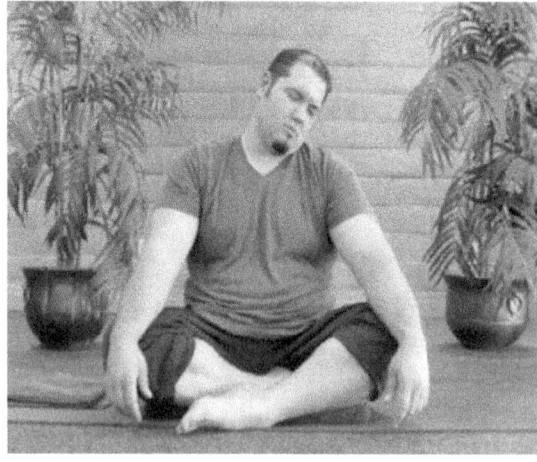

Lean the ear to the shoulder. Now lower the chin to chest. Keep this a full circle.

Do repetitions of 4 on each side.

HIP ROCK

Unlocks Tight Hips, Messages Hip Joints

Tones Buttock Muscles

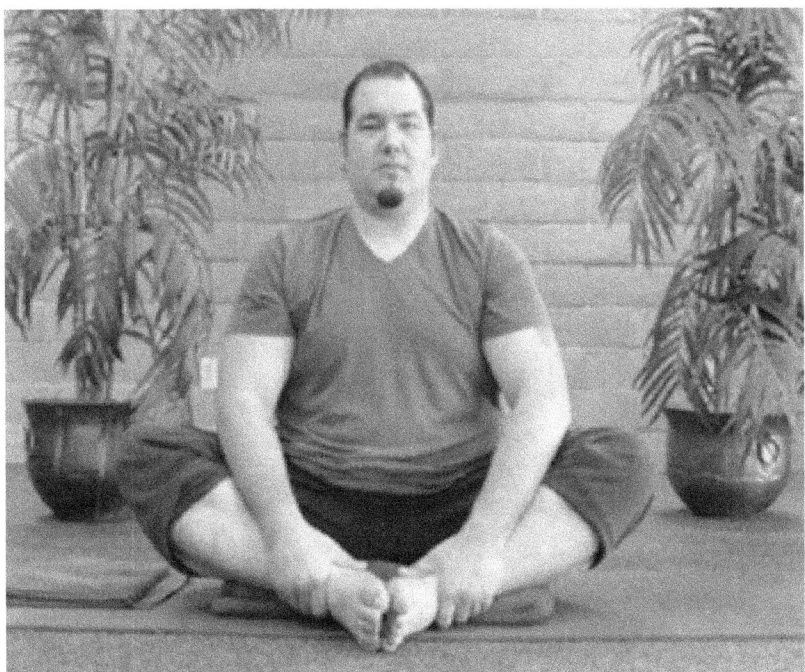

Begin by sitting with the souls of the feet together. Shift your weight to the left and place your right, bent leg at a 90 degree angle from the midline of the body. The sole of the left foot is aligned with the right hip flexor. Rest the left hand, beside your body.

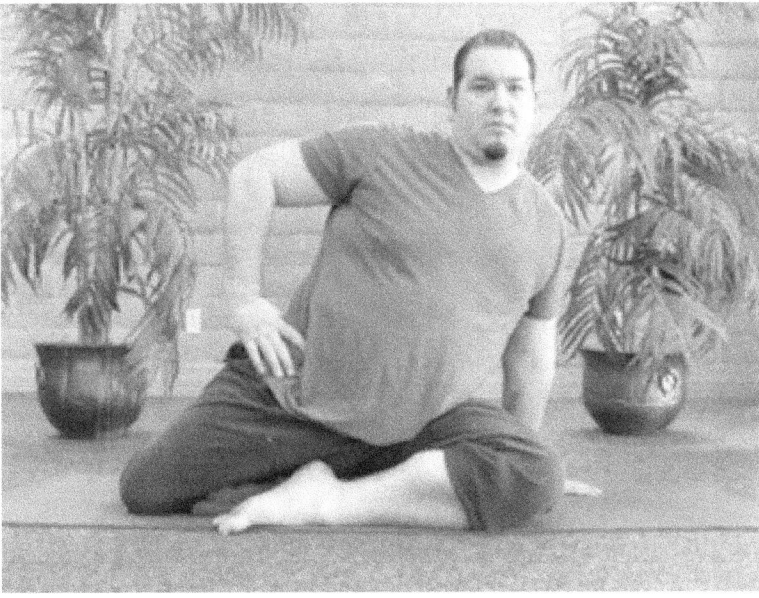

Place the hand on your right hip bone and slowly rock the hip front, contracting the gluteus (buttock muscles).

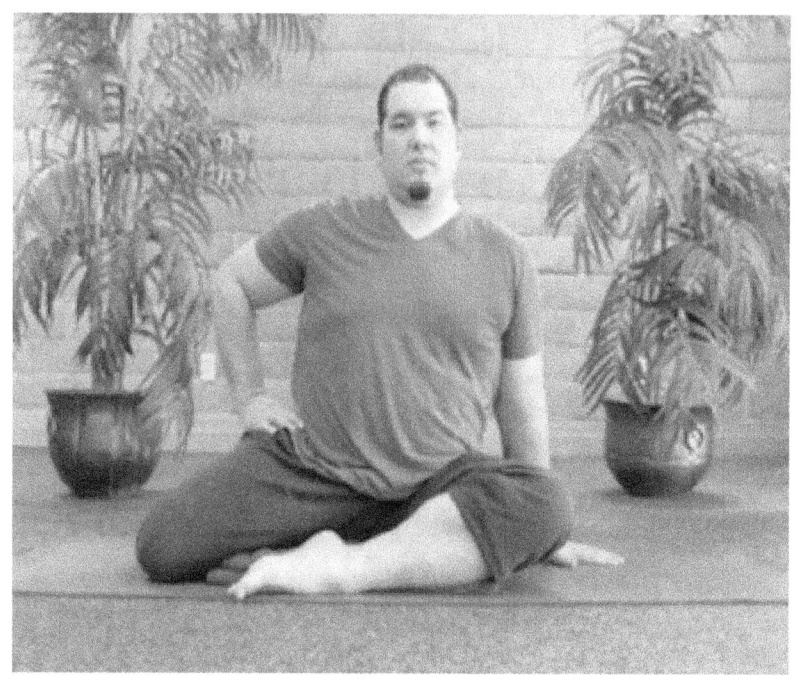

Release the buttocks and ease the sit bones as far back down to the floor as possible.

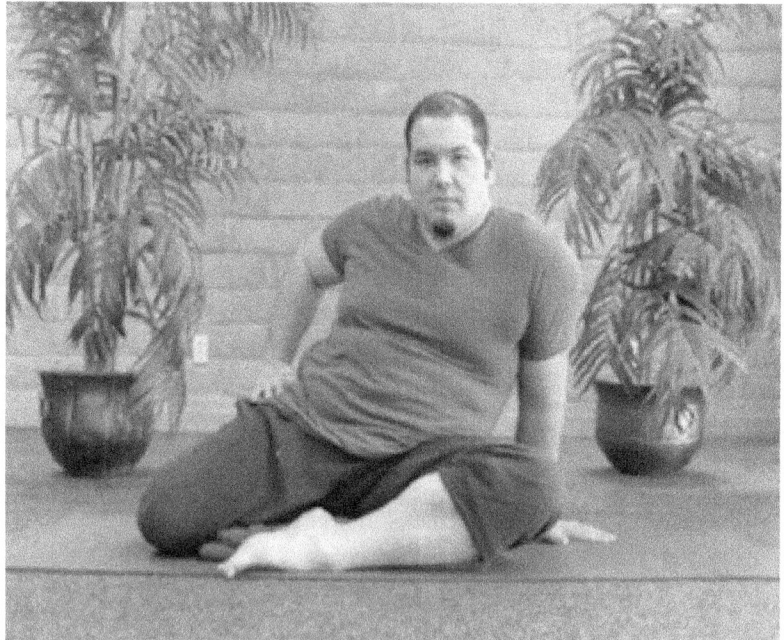

You should feel a deep opening in the rotation of the hip joint in both directions.

Repeat 8 x's

Again sit with the soles of the feet together and repeat the sequence on the other side.

OPEN LEG STRETCH

Unlocks the Hip Flexors, Calves and Hamstrings

Stretches Adductors and Strengthens the Back

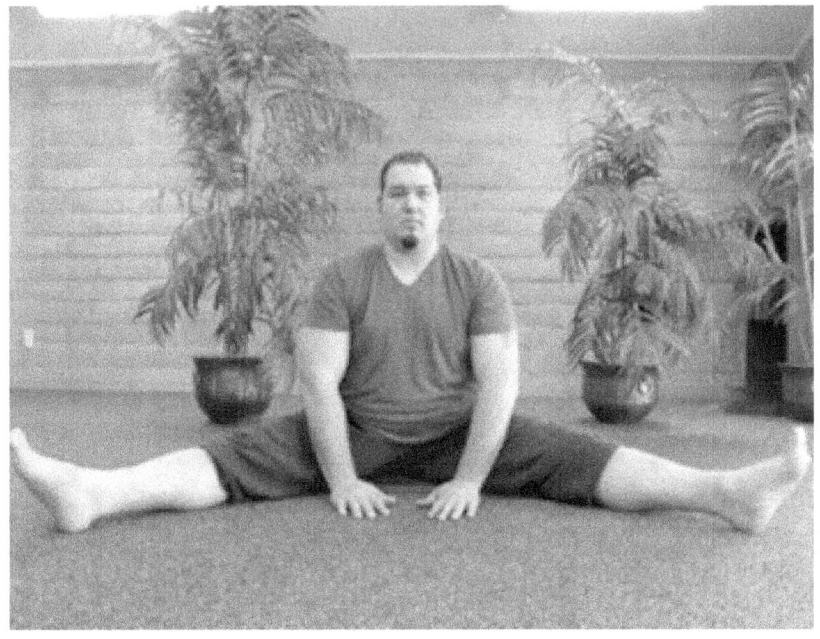

Sit with the legs open as far apart as comfortable. If the back and hamstrings are tight, bring the legs in closer together. Keep the spine tall.

*Avoid rounding the back. Also, be mindful that the legs don't roll inward. Keep them in a long line from the body, letting the energy come all the way out through the feet.

Place the hands on the floor in front of you and extend the legs. Flex the feet.

Lift up and rotate the pelvis forward slightly but do not allow the legs to rotate. Hinge forward if flexibility allows.

Feel a lovely openness in the hip flexors, back of legs and out through the feet.

Hold for count of 15

GENTLE SPINAL TWIST

Opens the Erector Spinae, Pectorals Muscles, Abdominals, Obliques, and Gluteus

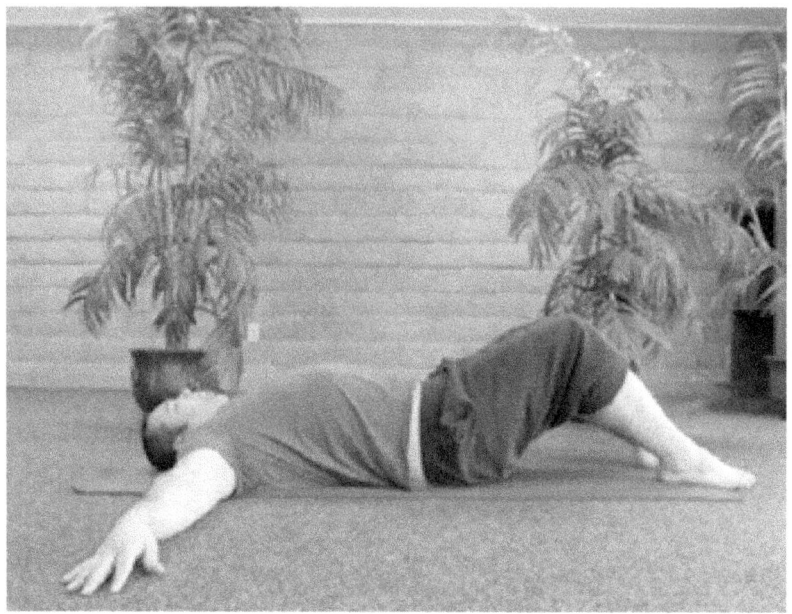

Lie on your back. Stretch both of your arms straight out to the sides in line with the shoulders.

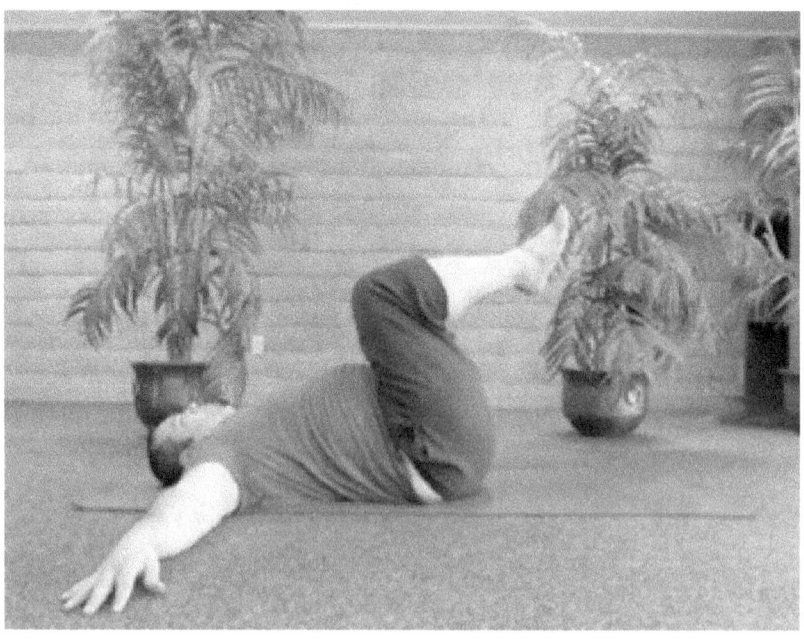

Bend your knees and bring them toward your chest.

Using your abdominals and with control, lower the legs slowly to one side.

*They do not have to come to the floor.

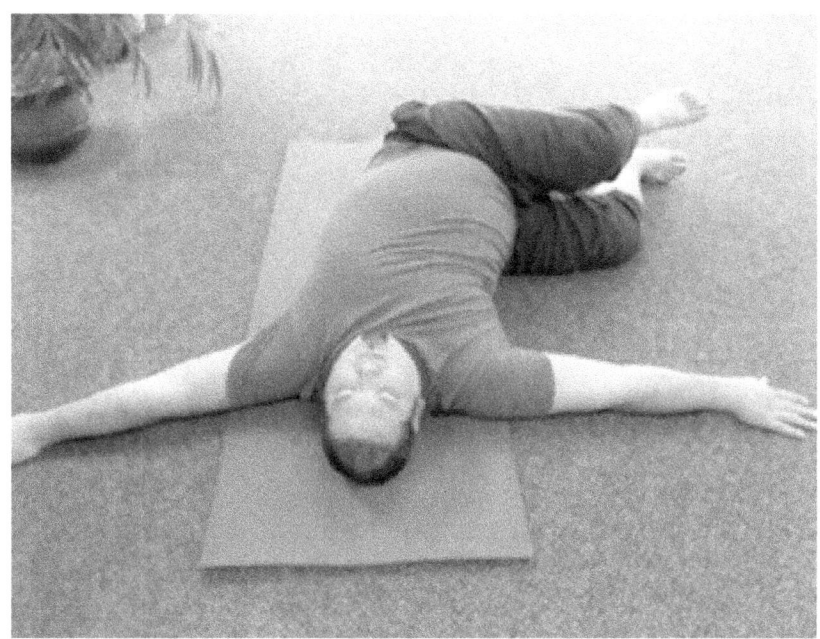

Breathe and allow the body to open without resistance. Hold for a count of 15.

Press the palms into the floor as you draw the knees into the center line. If you feel any strain at this point, lift the top leg first and then follow with the other leg.

Ease the legs toward the other side of the floor, rest and breathe. Hold for a count of 15.

Bring legs in toward the center or bring them in one at a time.

Hug the knees into the chest and release the spine.

*If you have restricted breathing when pulling your knees to the chest, separate your knees slightly.

RECLINING TAILBONE SCOOP

Works the Lower Quadrant of the Abdominals

Releases the Lower Back

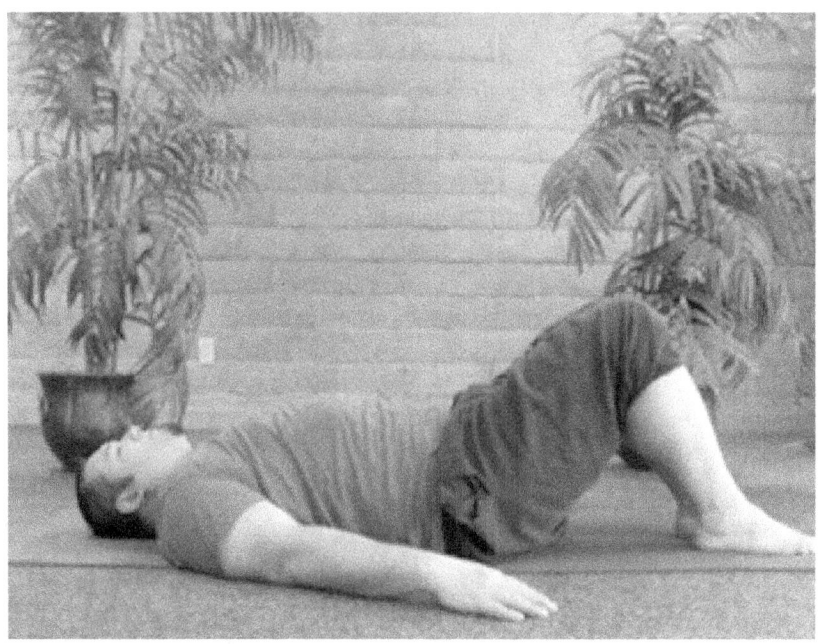

Lie on your back with your arms comfortably at your sides. Bend the knees so that the feet rest fully on the floor. Leaving the lower back on the floor, scoop the pelvis in. Use your abdominals without squeezing the buttocks. Keep the neck neutral and the shoulders resting on the floor. Do 16 controlled contractions with an equally controlled release.

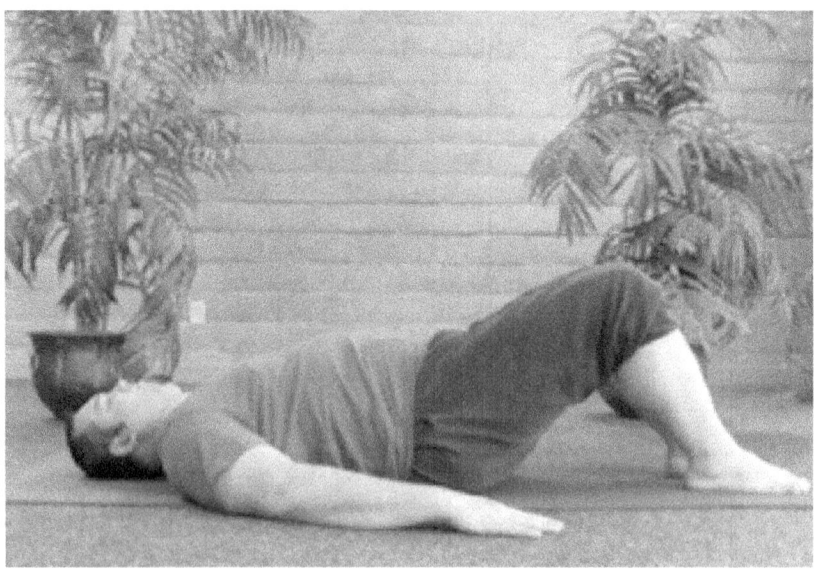

SUPER AB REHAB

Firms Entire Rectus Abdominis

Protects Lower Back and Strengthens the Neck

Begin by lying on the floor. Bend the knees so the soles of the feet rest comfortably on the floor. Place the hands behind the head. Press the tailbone toward the floor. Scoop the buttocks under, contracting the lower abs. Using the strength of your abdominals, exhale and lift the head a few inches off the floor. Slowly release the lower abs and then the upper abs. Repeat 5 x's with control.

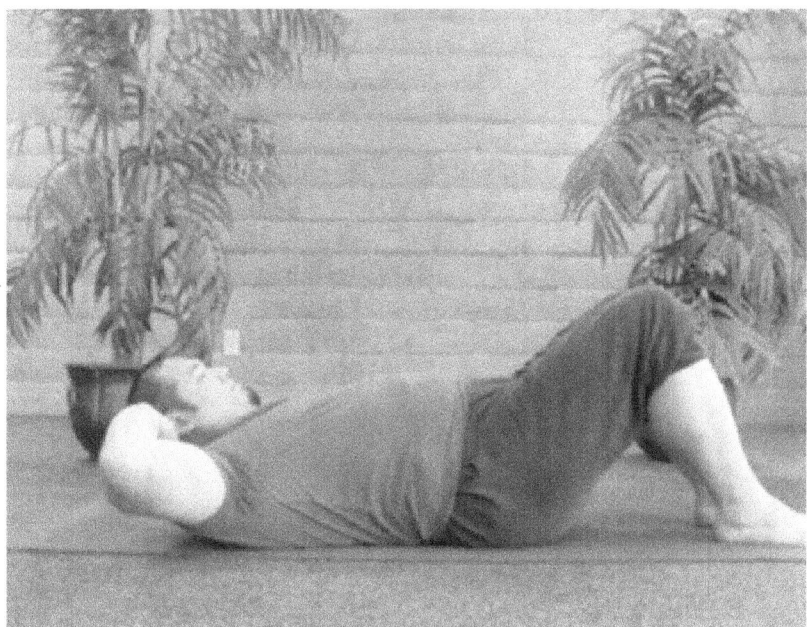

Contract the lower and upper abs together. Slowly release together.

Repeat 5 x's.

Do not strain. It's not how high you lift but how well you utilize the muscles.

STANDING FORWARD FOLD

Lengthens the Spinal Muscles, Stretches the Piriformis, Hamstrings and Calves

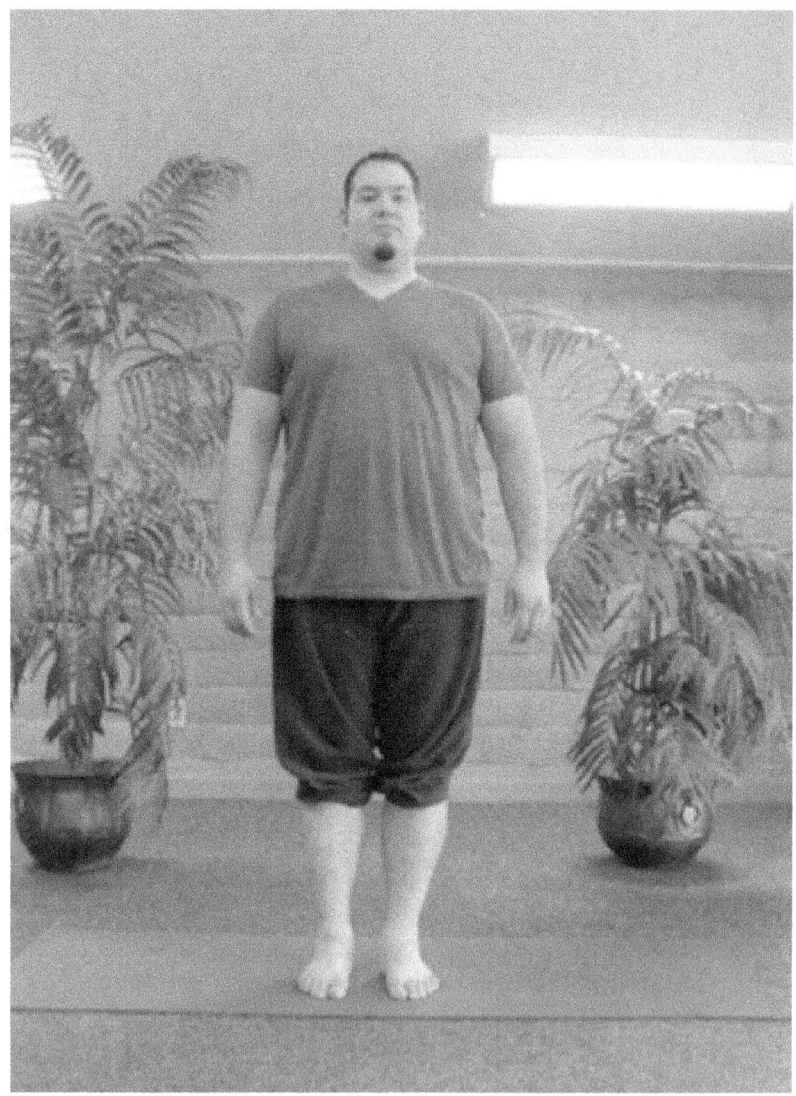

Stand with the feet inside the shoulders.

Bend the knees and roll down.

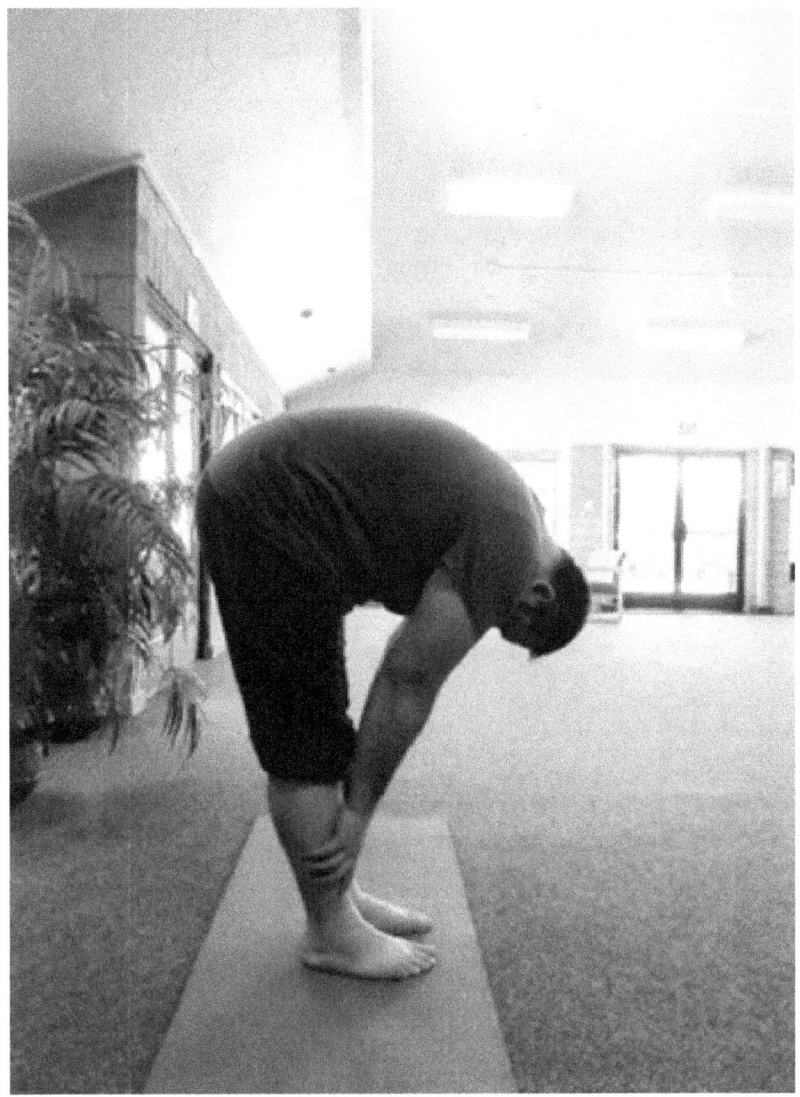

You may place your hands on your shins or on the floor.

Breathe through the back gills, letting the stretch expand the spine.

Hold for a count of 15.

*For tight hamstrings bend the knees.

To come up, contract your hamstrings (the back of the legs) and your buttock muscles. This will spare any strain in the lower back. Take a moment and take a breath.

STANDING FORWARD TRIANGLE

Releases Hamstrings, Calves, Buttocks

Unlocks the Hip Flexors

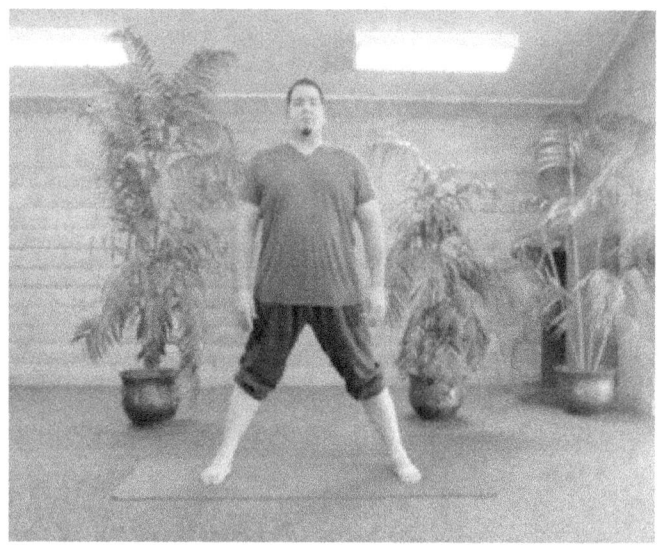

Stand with the feet wider than shoulder width. Feel each part of the foot connect with the floor and keep them parallel.

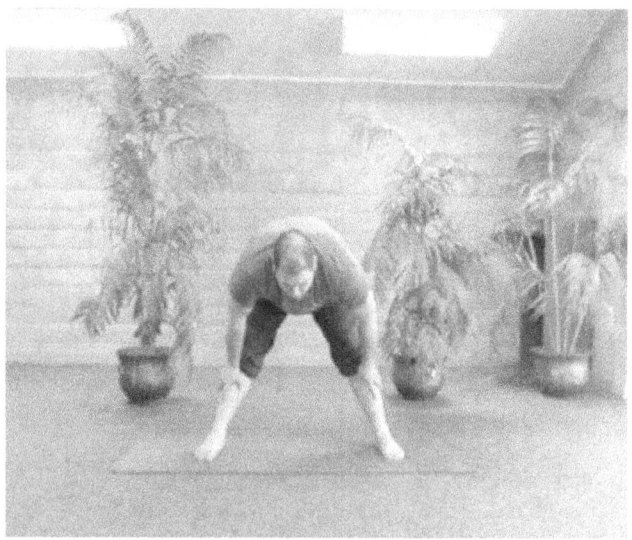

Using the buttock and hamstring muscles come forward and rest hands either on the shins or the floor.

*If hamstrings are tight, bend the knees.

Relax and let the upper body hang as much as possible. If you're really tight, you may find the stretch in the spinal muscles also.

*Remember you should feel a good stretch but no pain. Allow the stretch to take form and wait. When the body is ready to let go, then do so. Hold for a count of 15.

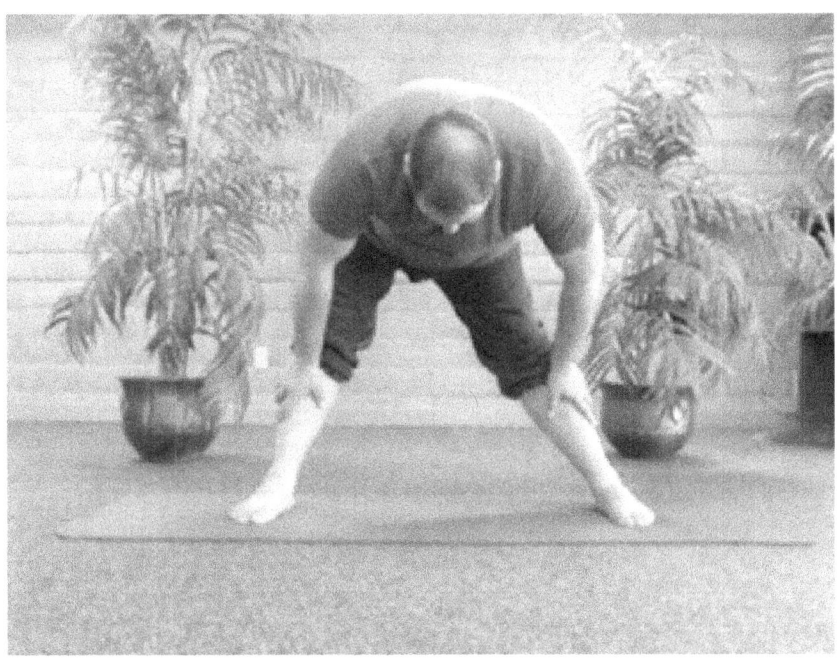

Now rock the hips back and forth slowly. The moment is small.

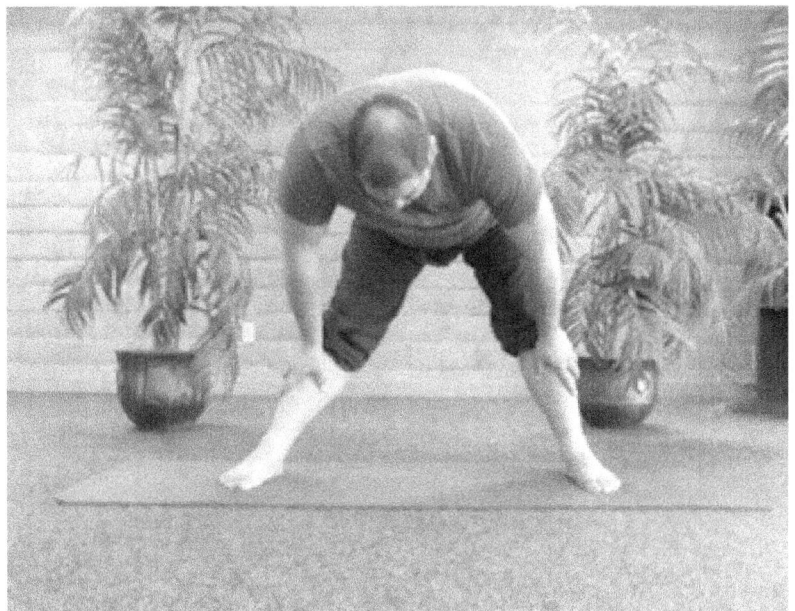

This rocking really opens and lubricates the joints within the hips. Rock 8 x's

To come out, contract the hamstrings and buttocks upon rising.

A note about micro tears. Micro tears occur when we push beyond our limits in a stretch before our bodies are ready to. In response, the muscle tears and creates scar tissue and additional inflammation. It causes pain, setting your progress back. This is why it is imperative to listen and respond to what your body is telling you. Telltale signs that you're pushing beyond your limit is constricted breath during a pose and tension instead of release. If you're cringing in pain, or discomfort you've definitely gone too far. Ease back and wait for your body to release.

STANDING HIP OPENER

Works the Quadriceps

Tones Adductors and Abductor Muscles

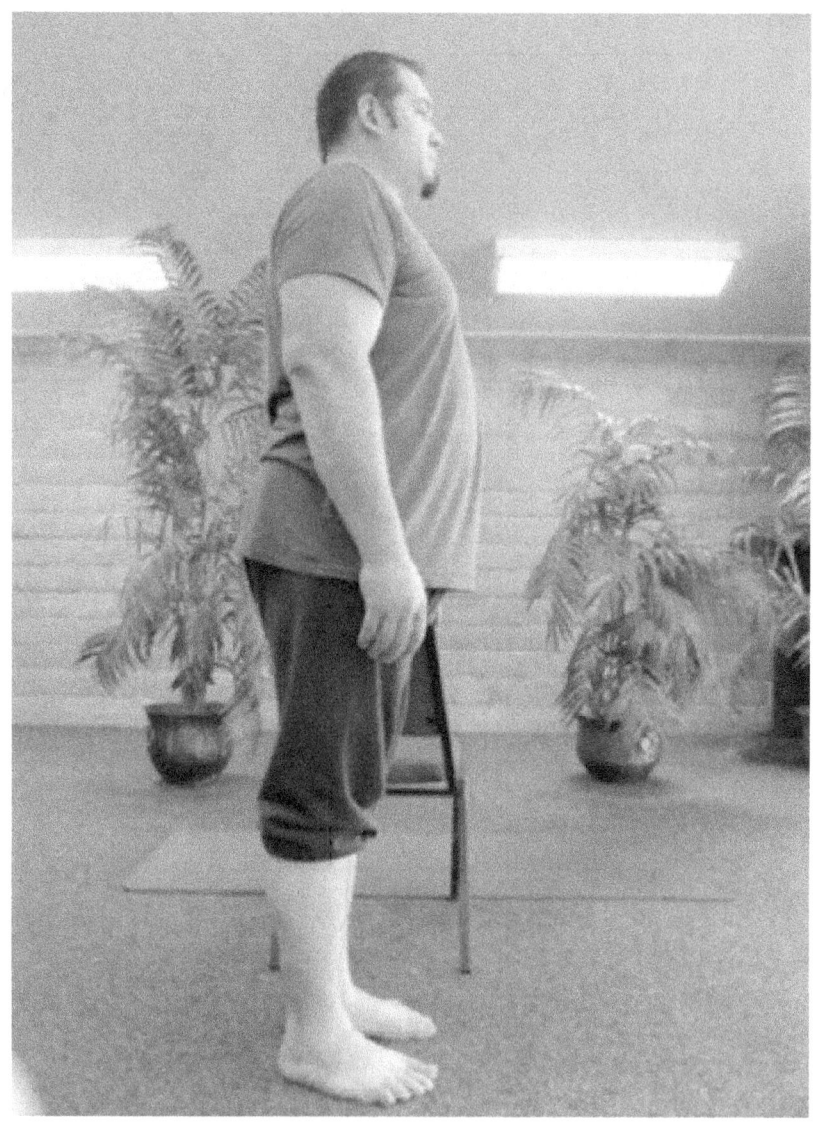

Standing with your feet inside your shoulders, hold onto a chair or stand with the support of a wall.

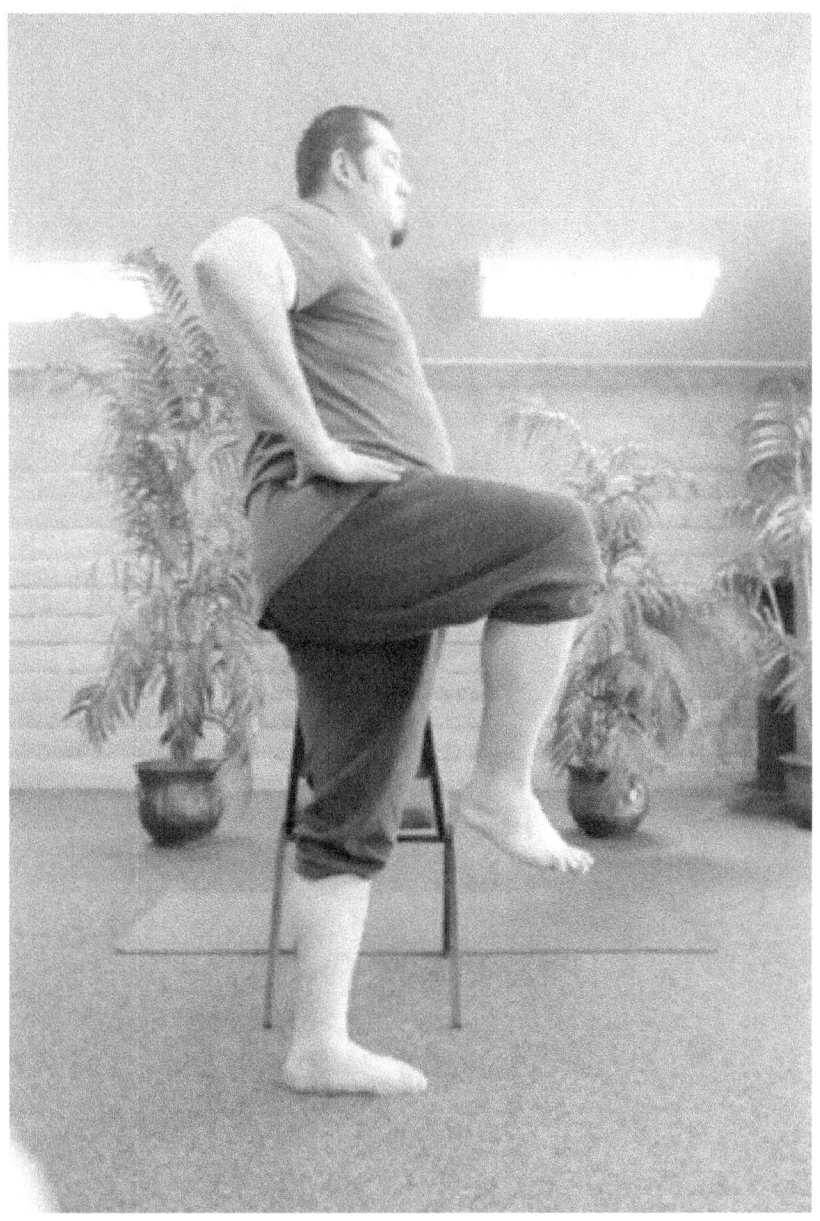

Bend the leg and lift it. Ideally you want to come up 90 degrees to the body line but if you cannot at this time just lift as high as comfortably possible.

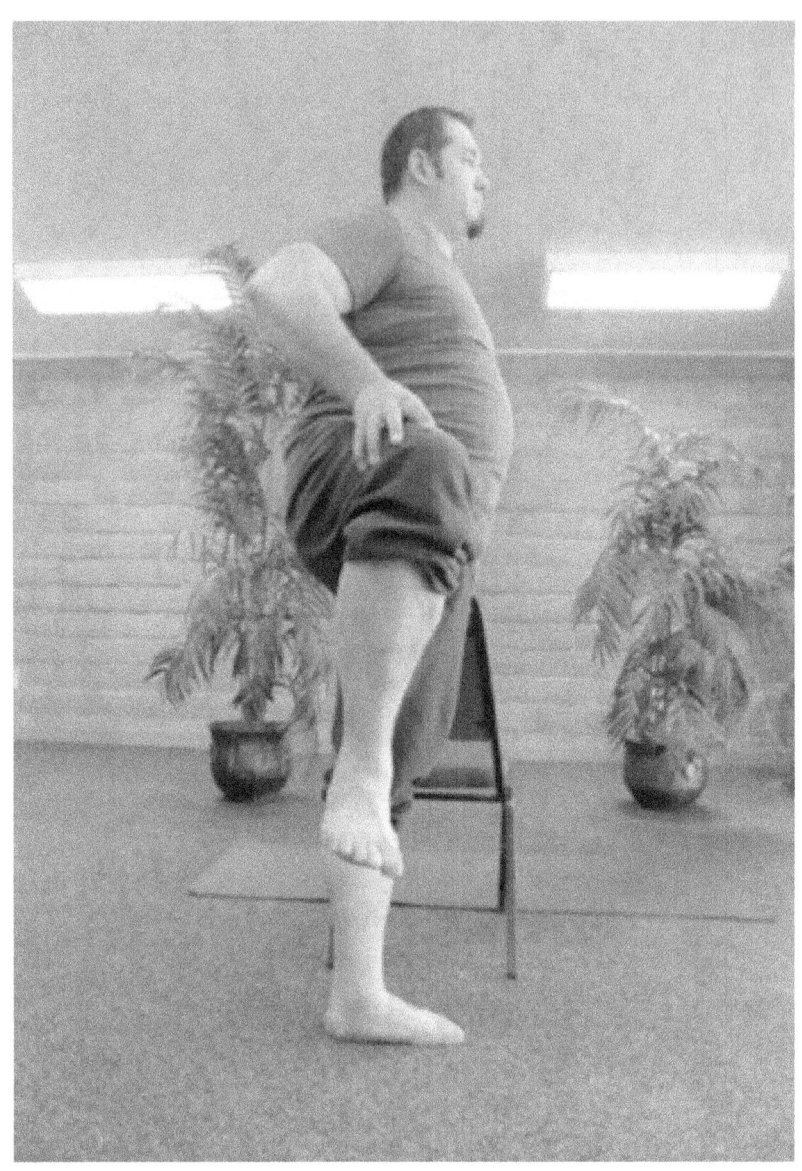

Let the free hand guide the leg out to the side and slightly back.

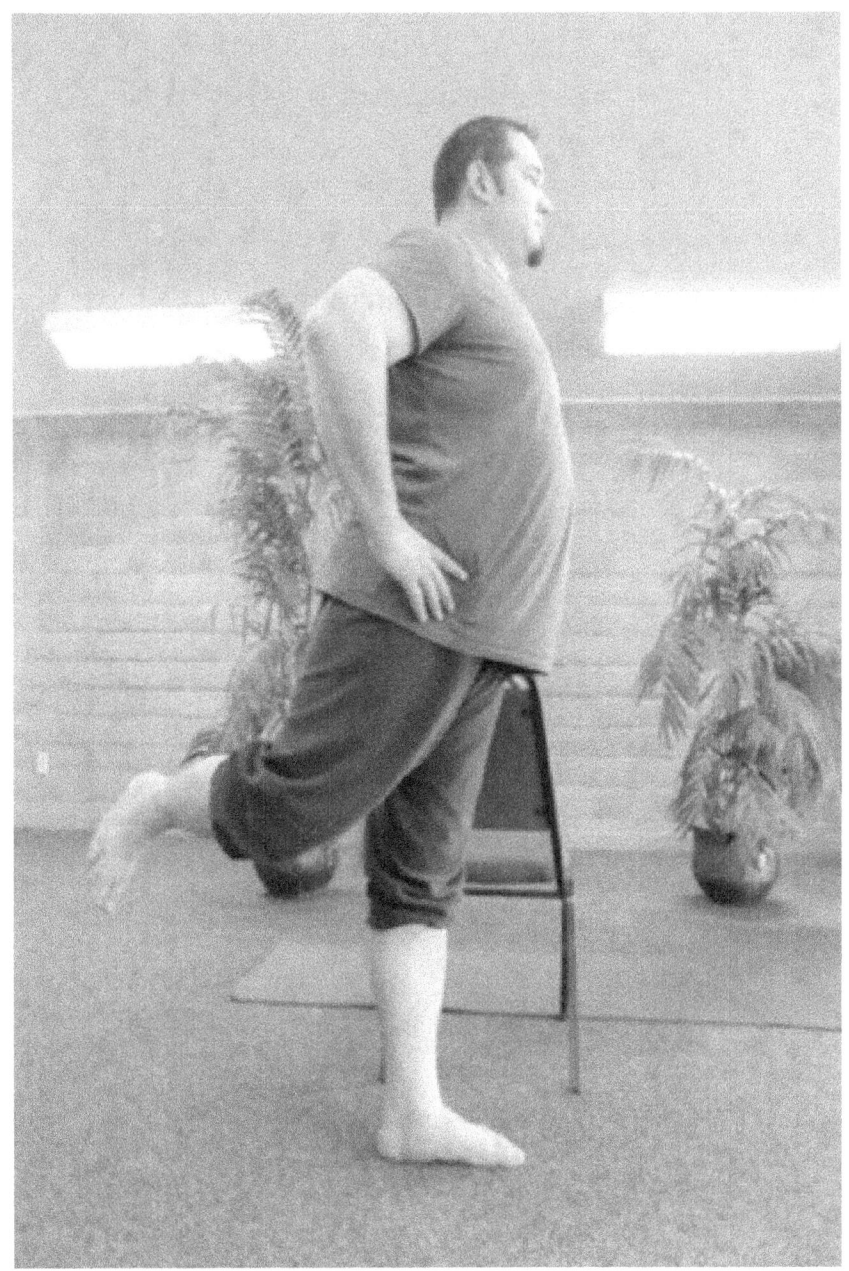

Lower the leg and bring it up to the front again.

This action forms a circle.

Do a repetition of 5 in one direction.

Now reverse directions. Begin by pushing the leg back then bring it out to the side.

Lift it front forming a circle in reverse.

Do a repetition of 5

ARM SEQUENCE

Stretches Shoulders, Chest, Biceps and Triceps

Shoulder Stretch

*These exercises can be done seated or standing.

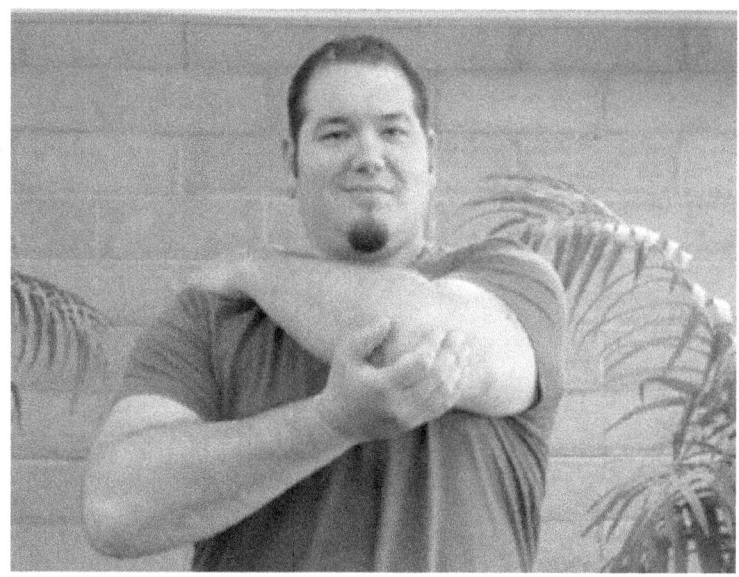

Begin by stretching the right arm out in front of you. Place your right hand on your left shoulder. Gently apply pressure with your left hand below the elbow. You should feel a stretch along the posterior deltoids (back of shoulder). You may also feel this around the shoulder blades also.

Hold for count of 15. Slowly release.

Repeat on the other side.

A note about chair sitting: Try to incorporate floor sitting or sitting on a balance ball every day. Sitting in a chair closes the hips, weakens the back and tightens the muscles. You may of course place a blanket or cushion beneath you if you're sitting on the floor. It's important to open and to keep our spines strong. Floor sitting or balance ball sitting can help strengthen those muscles that weaken in chairs.

Triceps Stretch

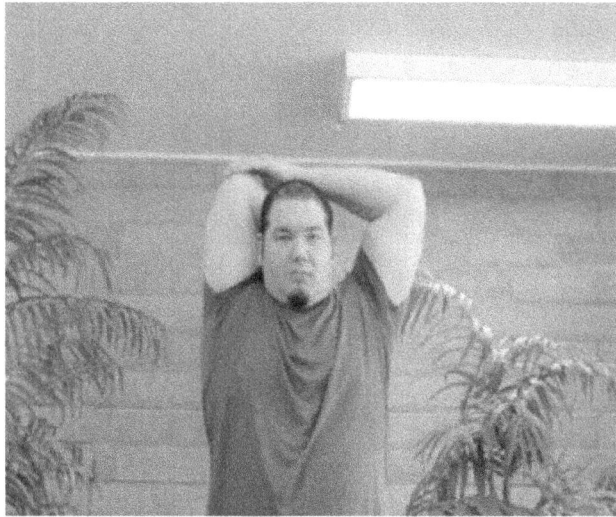

Bend the elbow, tuck the chin slightly downward and place the hand down the back of the head.

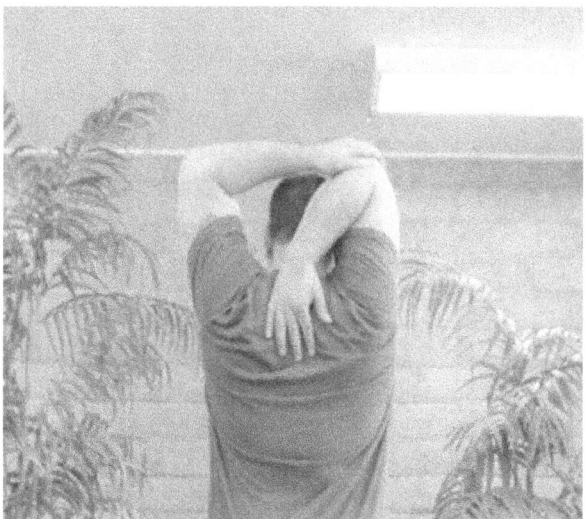

With the other hand apply gentle pressure to the elbow, feeling a nice stretch along the triceps.

If you are really tight, drop the chin a little more.

Don't give up. It's important that we create as much balance in our body as possible.

Note:

Over use or stretching of certain muscles while ignoring others, causes muscular overload. This guarantees inflammation due to a burden of stress. One muscle cannot do the work of another but it will try to make up for it when we aren't balanced. More injuries happen this way Pay attention to where you're tight or feel restriction and make a commitment to work on this part of you, giving yourself great care and patience.

CHEST STRETCH

Stand with your feet a comfortable distance apart.

Keeping the spine tall, soften the knees.

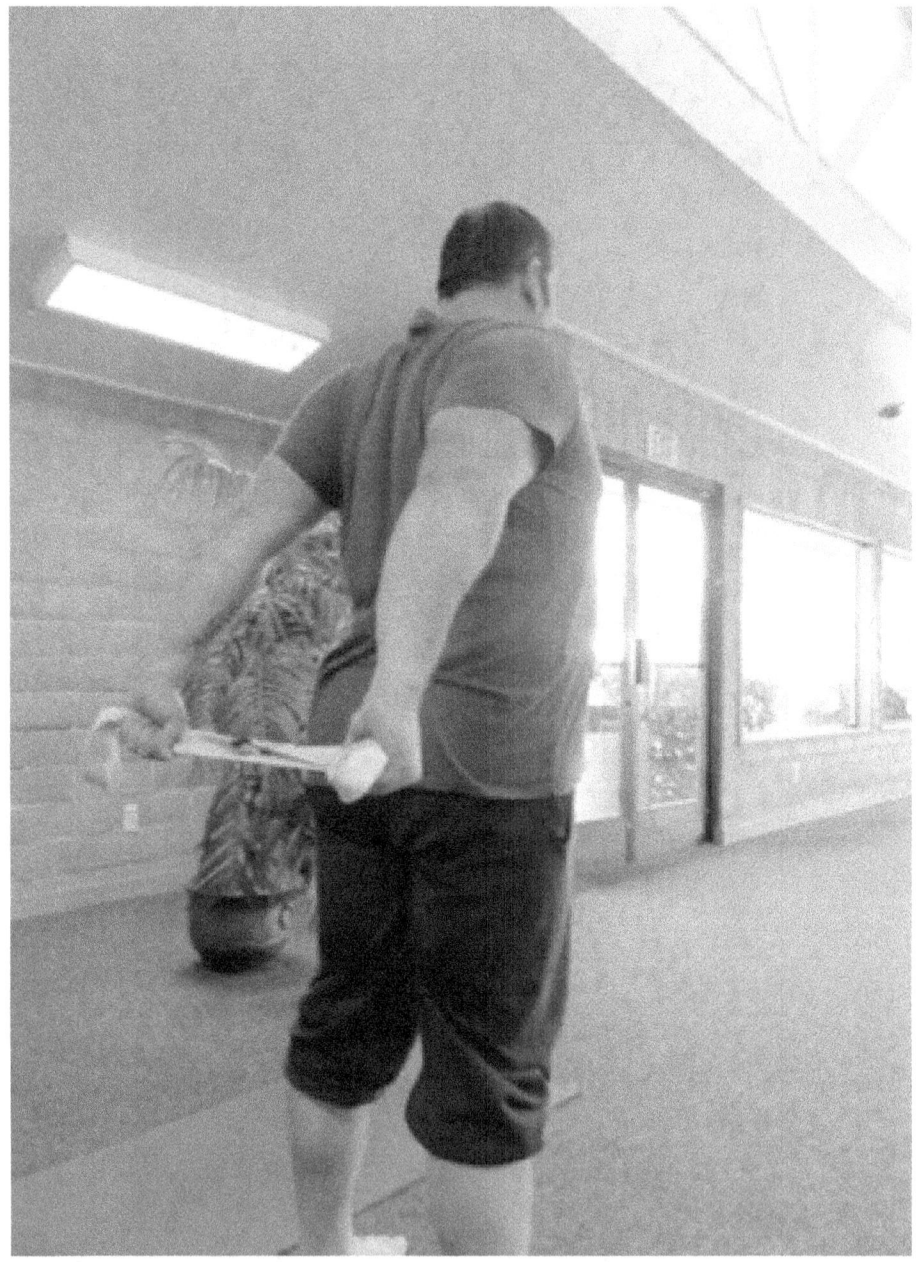

Reach behind you and interlace your hands by drawing your shoulder blades down your back.

If you're very tight use a towel or strap as shown.

There will be a slight arch in the back but do your best not to hyperextend.

Hold for a count of 15.

EASY DOWNWARD DOG

Strengthens Biceps, Triceps, Deltoids, Latissimus Dorsi, Gluteus Muscles

Lengthens and Strengthens Hamstrings, Calves, Quadriceps and Feet

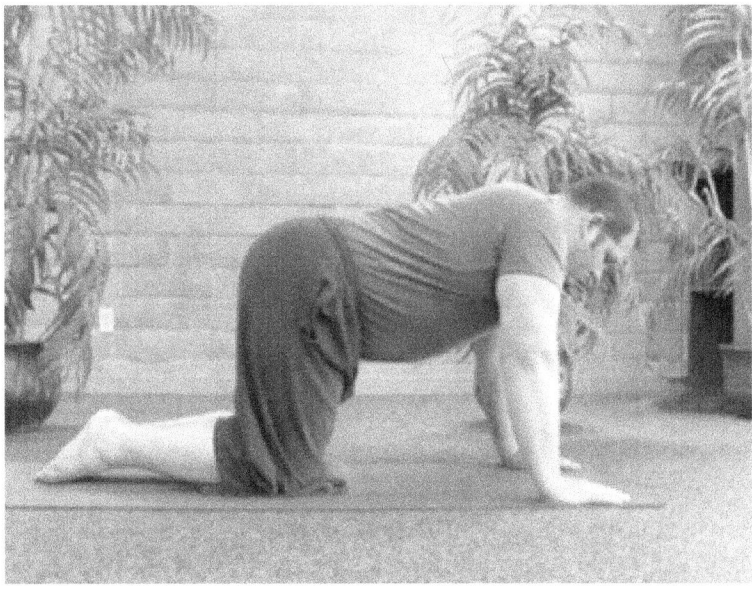

Start in tabletop position. You may place a towel beneath the knees for extra comfort.

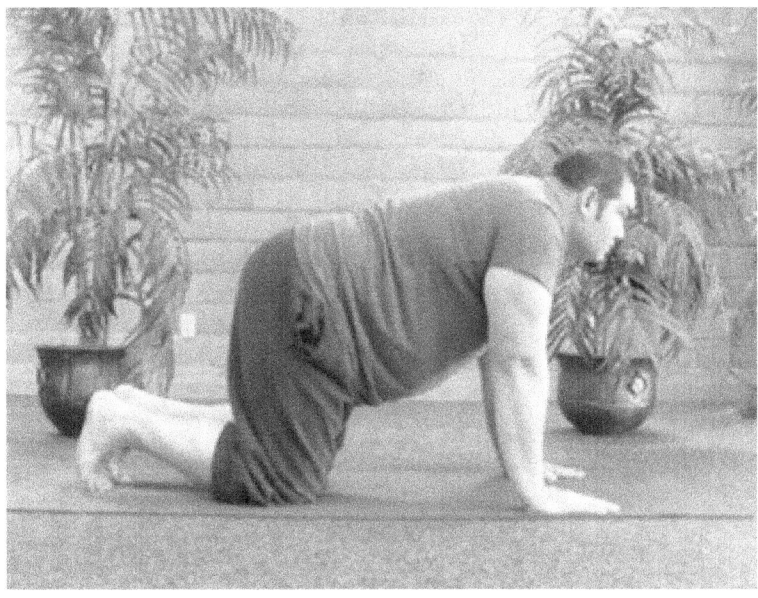

Curl the toes under and feel sturdy in the hands and shoulders.

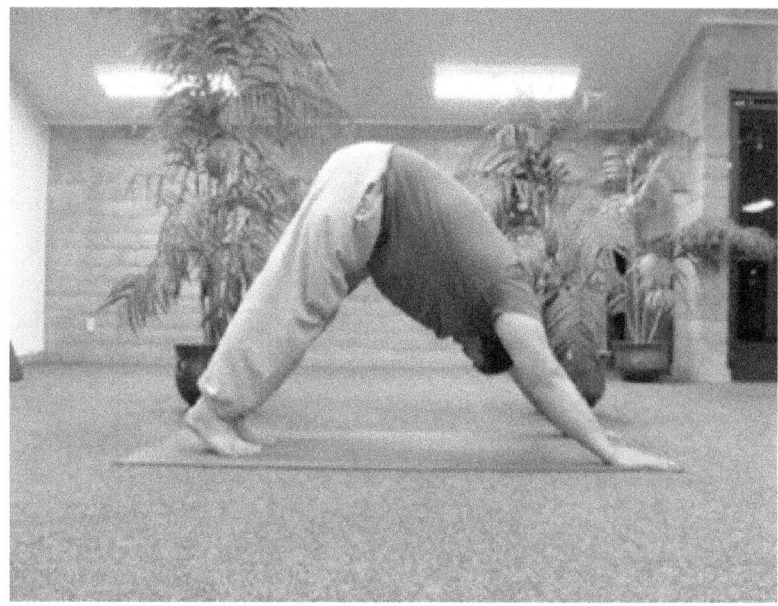

Lift the buttocks up by pushing through the strength of the shoulders, upper back and arms. Use the abdominals to maintain core balance. Now keeping the knees bent try and draw the abdomen to meet the knees. They won't touch necessarily. But this will allow the back to flatten and the tailbone to rotate upward.

(If you had an imaginary ball placed on the base of the tailbone it would ride right down the spine and fall off the crown.)

Feel the stretch in the back of the legs. Straighten the legs only until you want to increase the stretch. Feel a radiant expanse along the buttocks and back of legs.

Hold and breathe deep for a count of 15.

Bend the knees and return to tabletop for a few breaths.

*This pose also restores balance, improving circulation to the heart and brain.

CAT AND COW

Strengthens the Wrists

Conditions the Spine

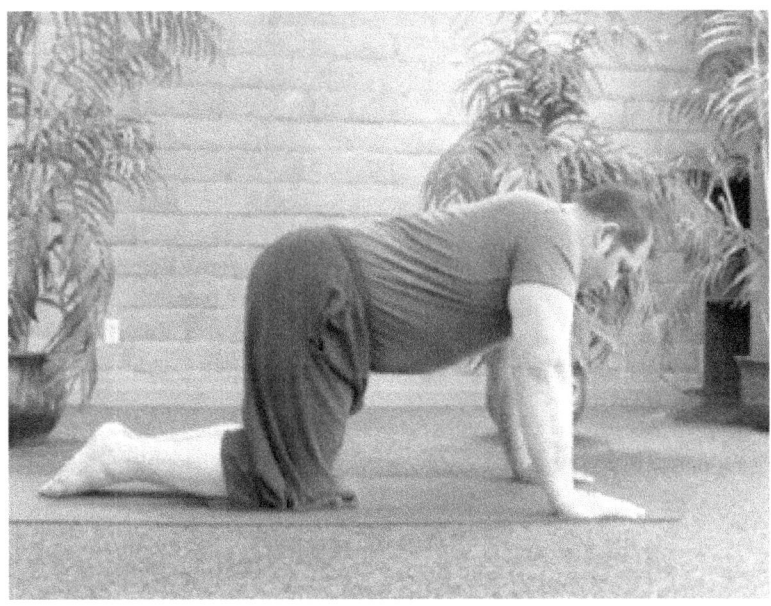

Come into tabletop position with the hands directly beneath the shoulders.

Keep the knees in line with the pelvis.

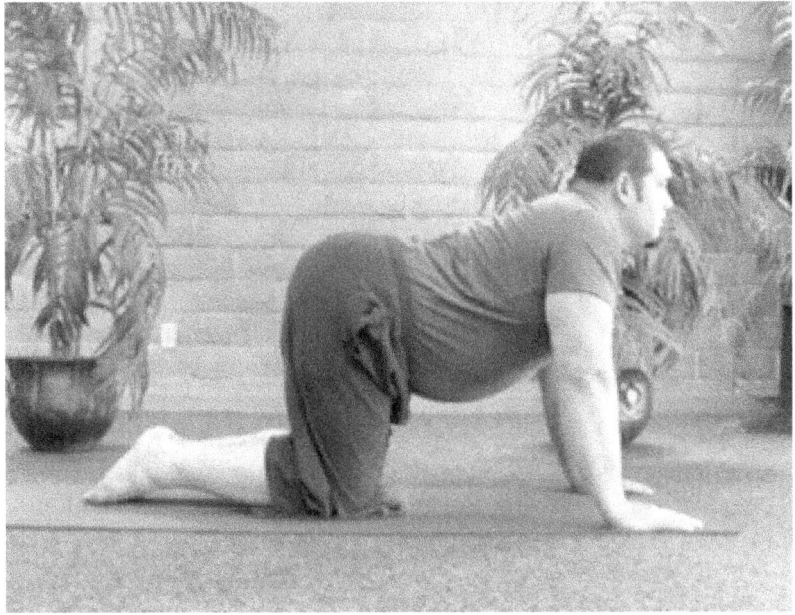

Take an inhale and arch the spine, allowing the neck to rise if it feels right.

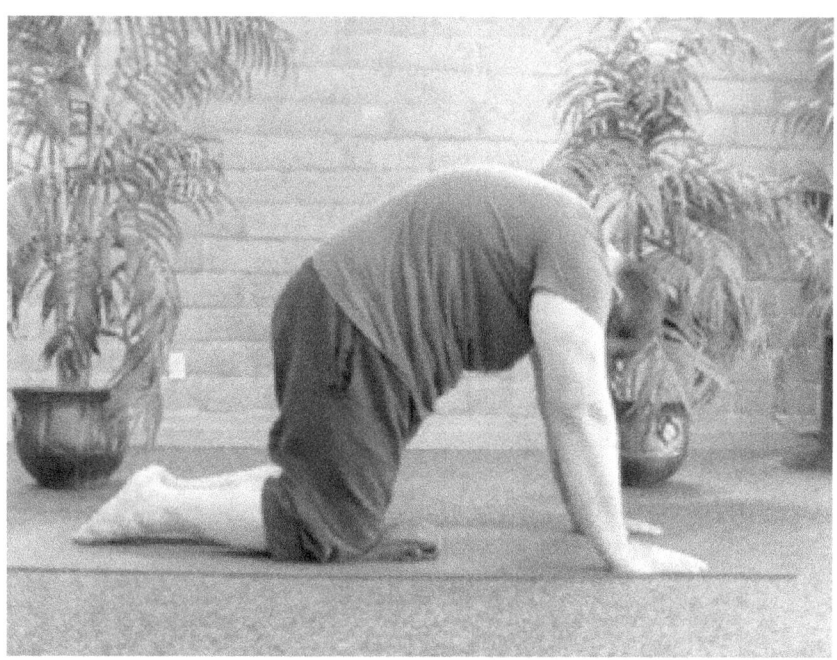

As you exhale curl the spine to the sky. Repeat going back and forth with a deep, calming breath. Repetition of 4 x's

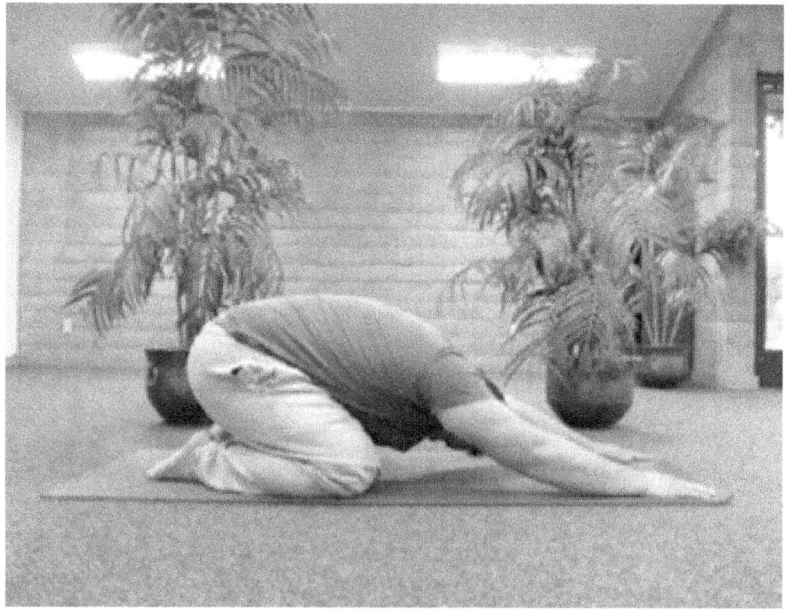

Separate the knees and push back into Child's Pose. It's not important that you rest your buttocks on your heels. Just go back as far as your flexibility will allow. This is a wonderful restorative pose. Stay here for a few breaths.

HIP FLEXOR STRETCH

Opens the Hip Flexors, Psoas Muscles and Quadriceps

Builds Strength and Balance

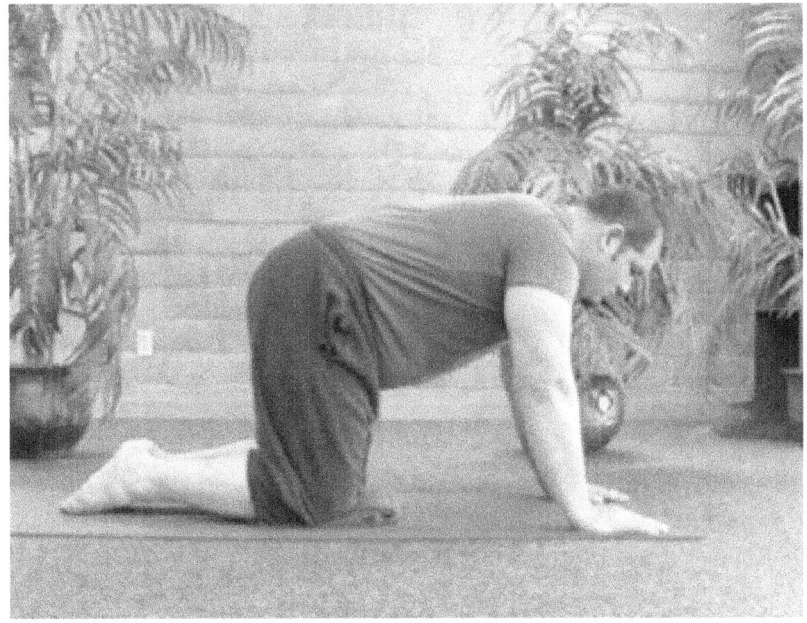

Start in table top position with a folded blanket or towel under the knees. Place the hands in line under the shoulders and the knees lined beneath the pelvis.

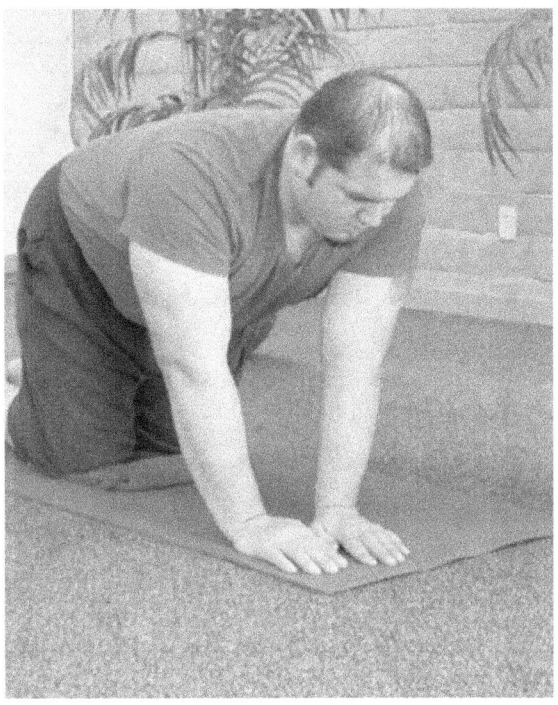

Take both hands and move them to the right side line.

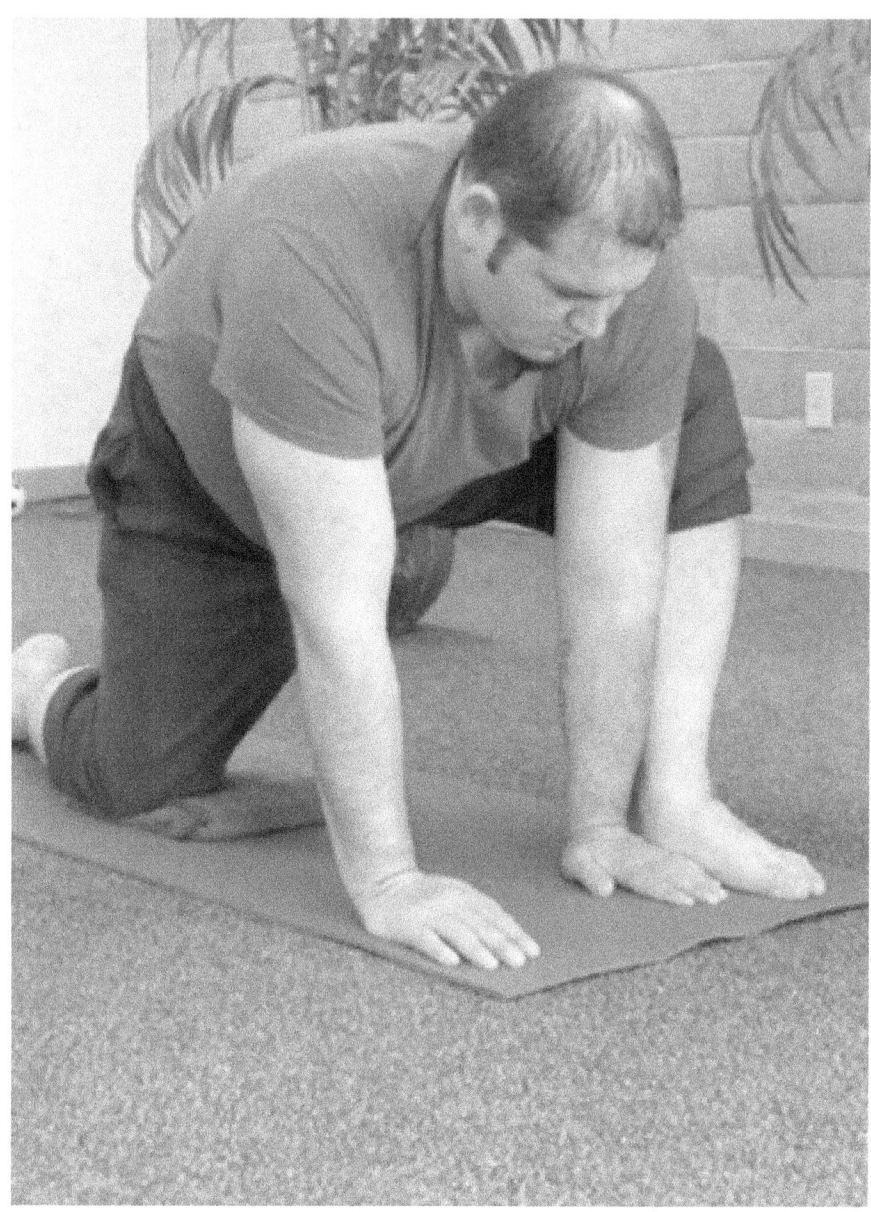

Step forward with the left foot.

*Keep the knee in line with the ankle. Pushing the knee beyond this point will put stress on the joint.

Line the left hand and arm close to the left foot. Feel secure between both arms. With awareness, place the left hand on the left thigh (not on the knee).

Raise the upper torso in line with the midpoint of the body.

Make sure the torso is not positioned too far back or too far forward.

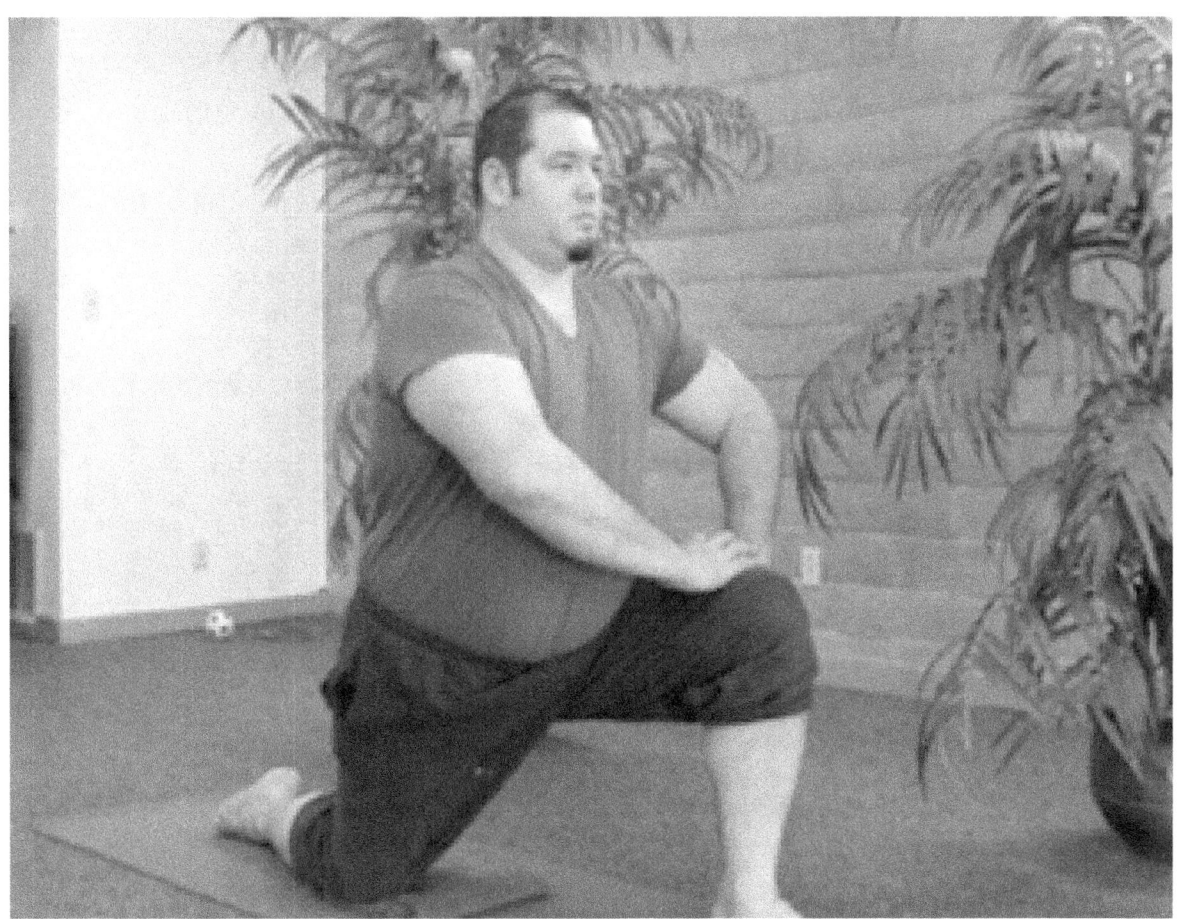

Press the hips down toward the earth keeping the spine strong and lifted.

Come down reversing the steps.

Repeat on the other side.

Hold for a count of 15.

Sit back on the heels or come into child's pose.

CALF STRETCH

Relieves Aches and Pains in the Calf Area

Begin in tabletop position. Walk hands to left side and step forward with the right foot as in previous exercise.

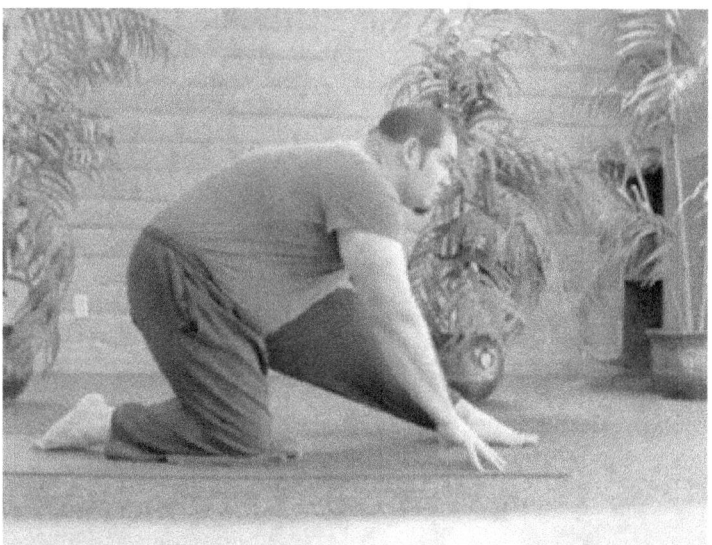

Reposition hands so that the leg sits between them. Shift your weight back.

*Do not sit down on the back leg. The front leg can remain bent if you feel tight.

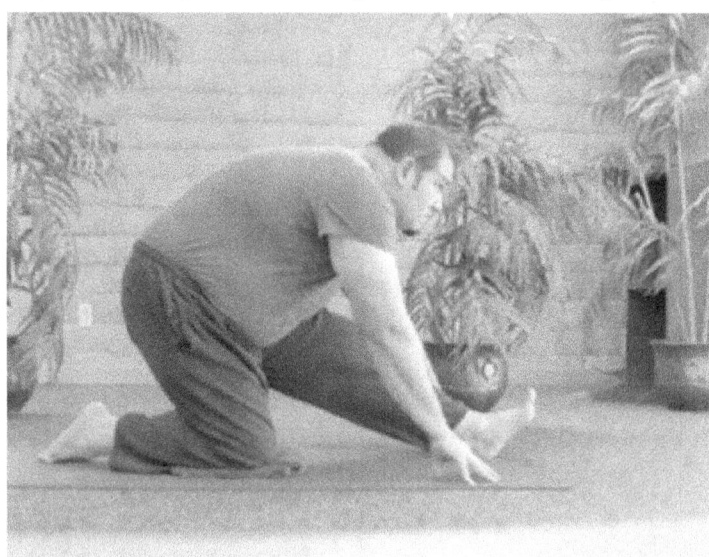

Draw the toes toward the floor feeling a stretch along the top of the foot, the calf and hamstring muscle. Hold for a count of 10.

This stretch can be challenging to some at first but if you practice it regularly, results will be seen quicker than you think.

Reverse the steps and repeat on the other side. Sit back on the heels if possible and relax for a few breaths.

SUPINE BUTTOCK STRETCH

Stretches the Gluteus Area

Releases Tension in the Lower Back

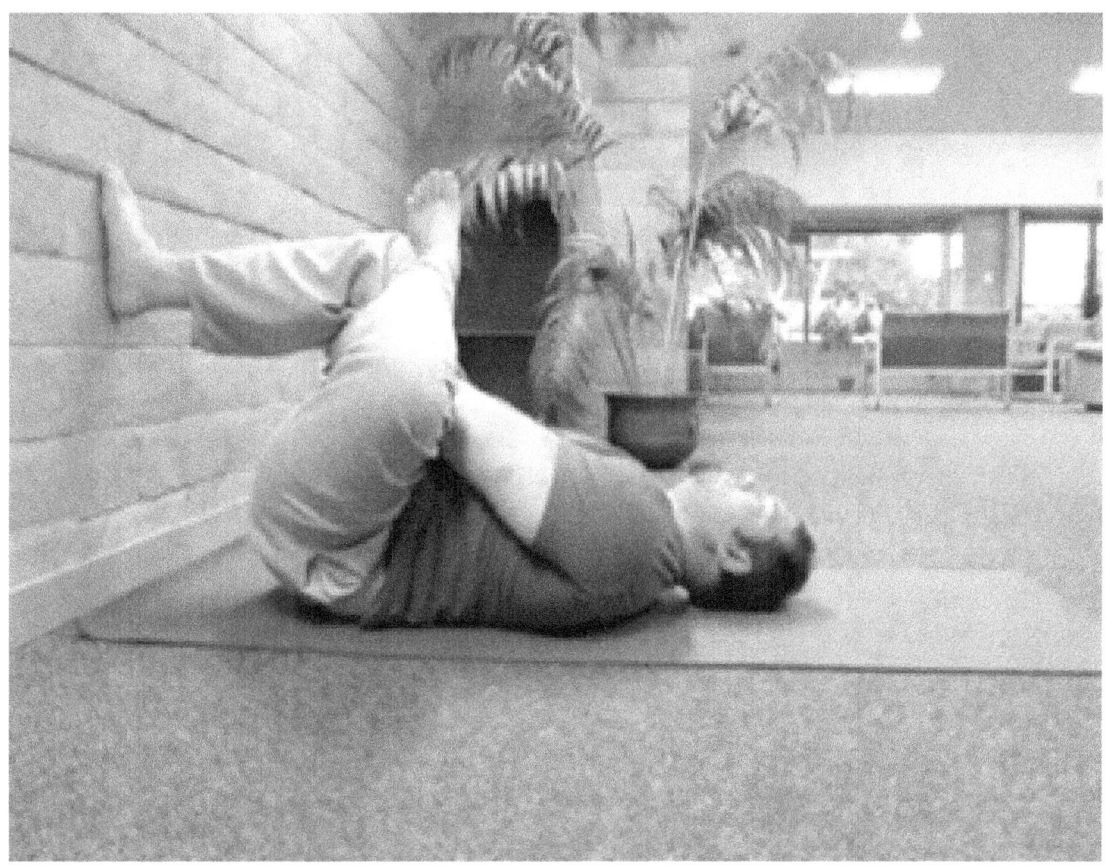

Lie on the floor close to a wall. Make sure your spine remains in contact with the floor at all times. Cross your right foot over your left thigh and place your left foot on the wall to assist in the stretch.

Repeat on the other side and hold for a count of 15.

*Keep the neck neutral.

Hold for a count of 15.

*This exercise does wonders for people who suffer with Sciatica.

RECLINING LEG STRETCH

Relieves Stress and Ache in Hamstrings, Lower Back and Calves

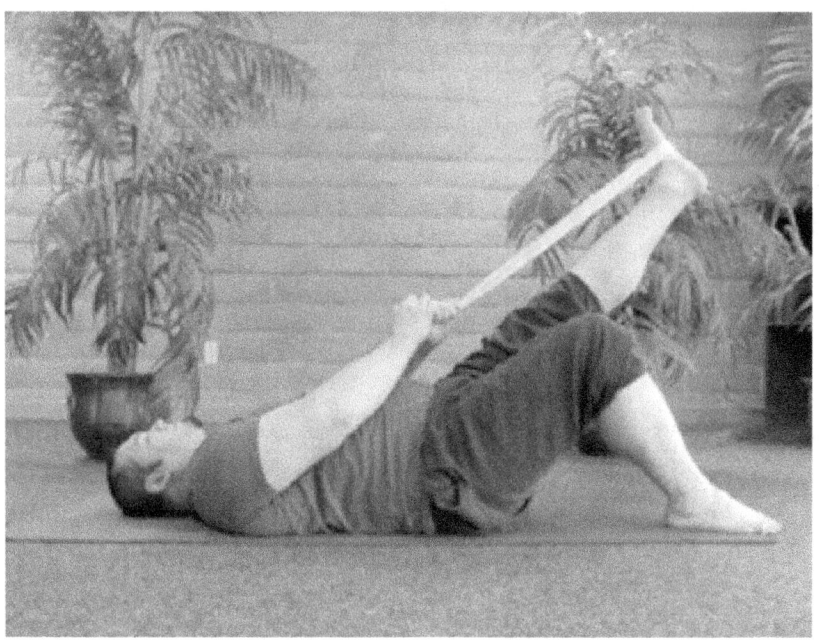

Lying on your back, bend your knees and place the feet on the floor. Make sure there is no space between your back and the floor.

Lasso a strap or towel around the sole of the foot and lift it to 45 degrees.

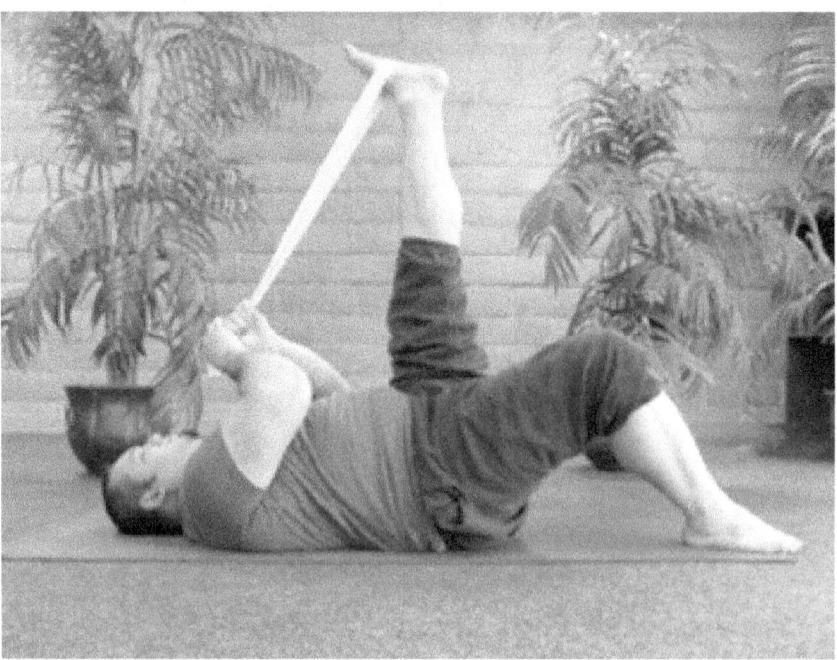

For an increased stretch lift it straight over the hip bone at 90 degrees. Breathe and hold this pose for a count of 15.

SIDE QUAD STRETCH

Stretches the Quads and Hip Flexors

Tones the Buttocks

Begin in a side lying position. Extend your arm beneath your head for balance.

Bend the bottom knee slightly and make sure the hips are stacked, so you're neither rocked forward or back. Bend the top leg and reach around to take hold of the foot or ankle.

Squeezing the buttocks tuck the pelvis slightly under and pull the foot toward your gluteus.

Feel a wonderful stretch in the front of the thigh.

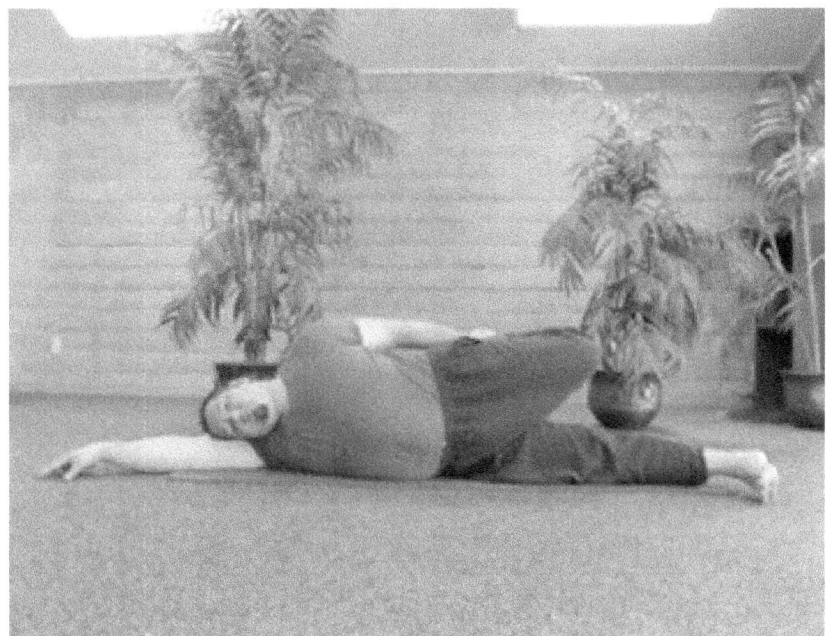

*It's important to make sure the bend in the knee stays parallel to the body. Otherwise you feel stress in the knee joint.

Hold for a count of 15.

Come up slowly. Shift to the other side and repeat. Hold for a count of 15.

You may lie on your back for a few breaths afterwards if you desire

KNEE REHAB

Strengthens the Knee and Massages the Joints

Increases Knee Lubrication

Come onto your back. Bend the knees and let the soles of the feet rest on the floor. Feel your spine connect to the earth. Let your arms rest at your sides with the palms down.

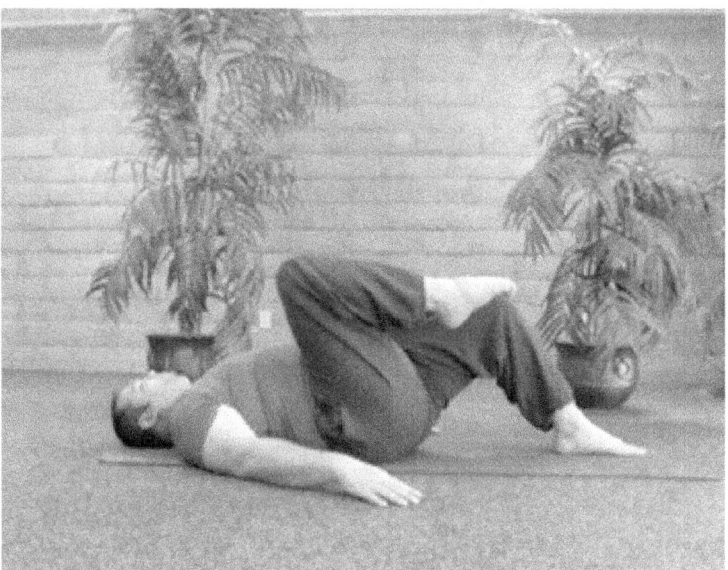

Begin by bending the knee in and pointing or elongating the foot.

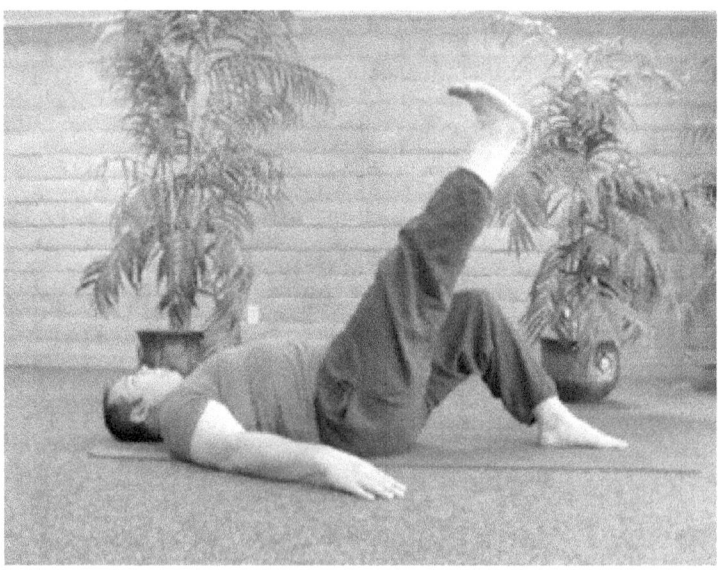

Lift the leg by straightening at the knee, about a 45 degree angle and flex the foot.

Draw the straight leg down with the heel.

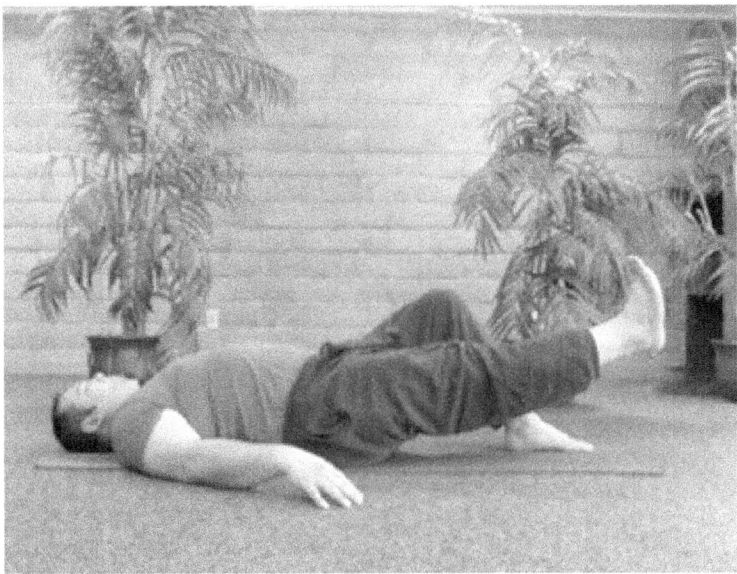

Repeat 5 x's

Reverse Process

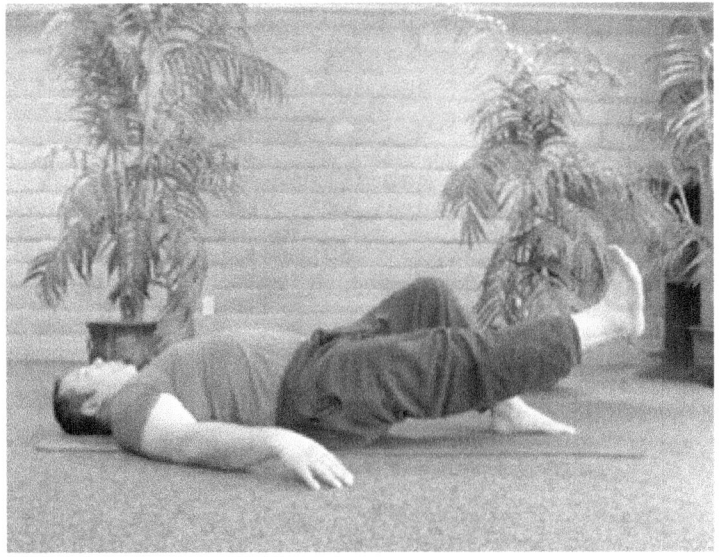

To reverse the process, lift the leg a few inches off the floor and flex the foot.

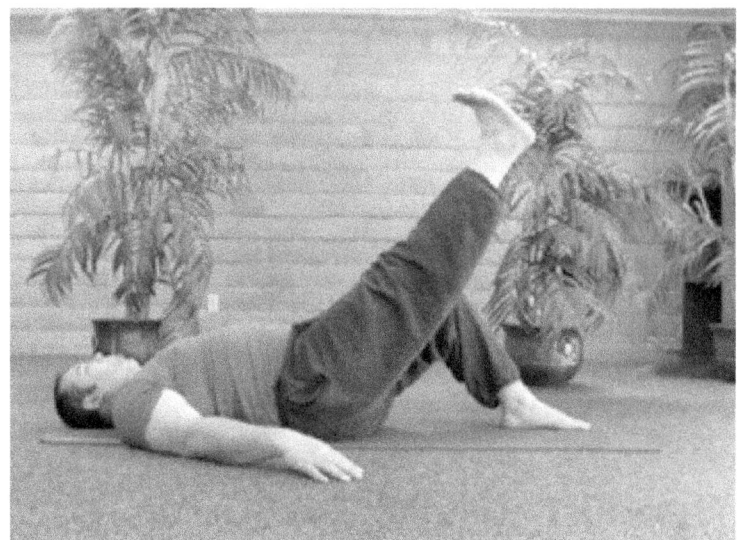

Raise the leg up toward the midline of the body.

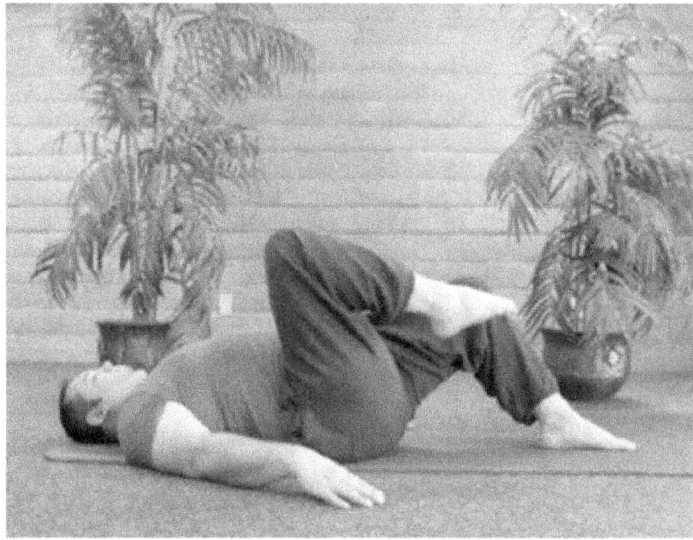

Bend the knee in toward the body as you point the toes.

Press the leg out with the heel and hover a few inches off the floor. Now bend the knee in and point the toes to repeat the sequence.

Repeat 5 x's

Adductor Extension

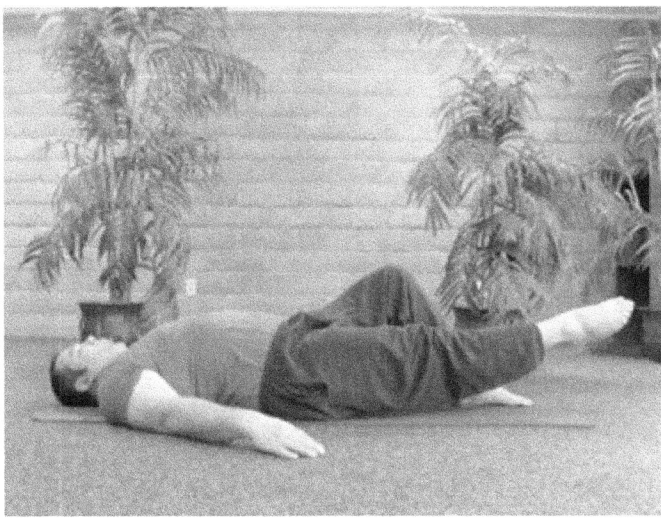

Lift the right leg an inch off the ground and keep it straight. Let the energy come out through the toes. Turn the leg out slightly, rotating from the hip. Brace yourself with your hands. Keep your abdominals firm to support you.

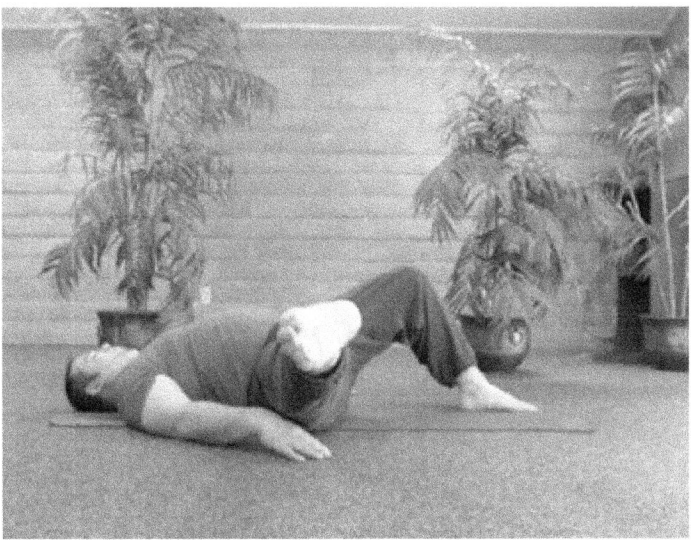

Extend the leg out from the midline of the body with a slow, controlled movement. Using your adductors (inner thighs) draw the leg back in.

Repeat 5 x's

Combination Sequence

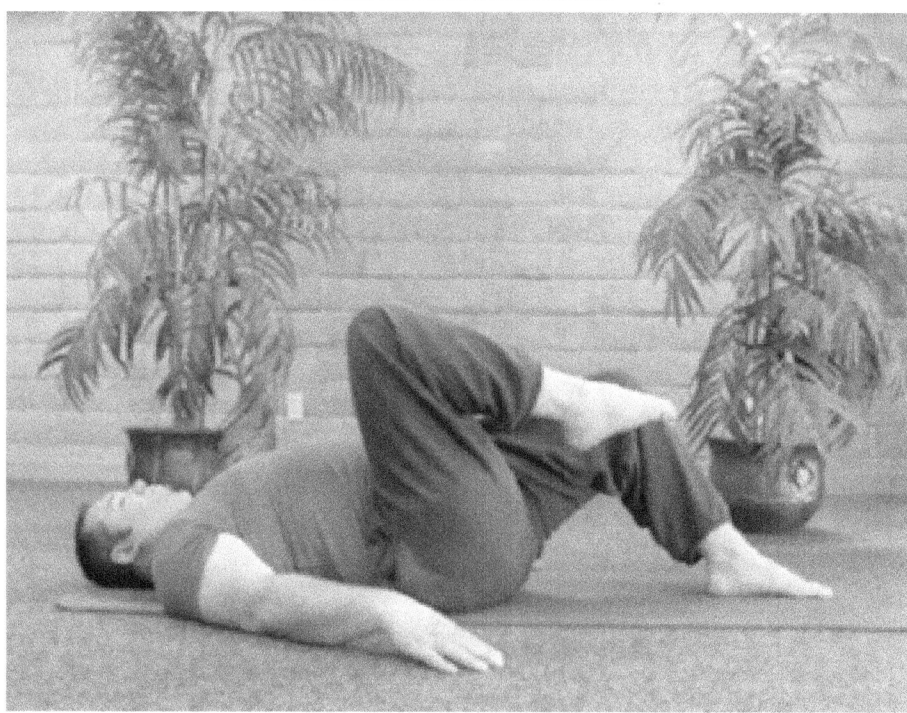

Bend the knee in and point the toes.

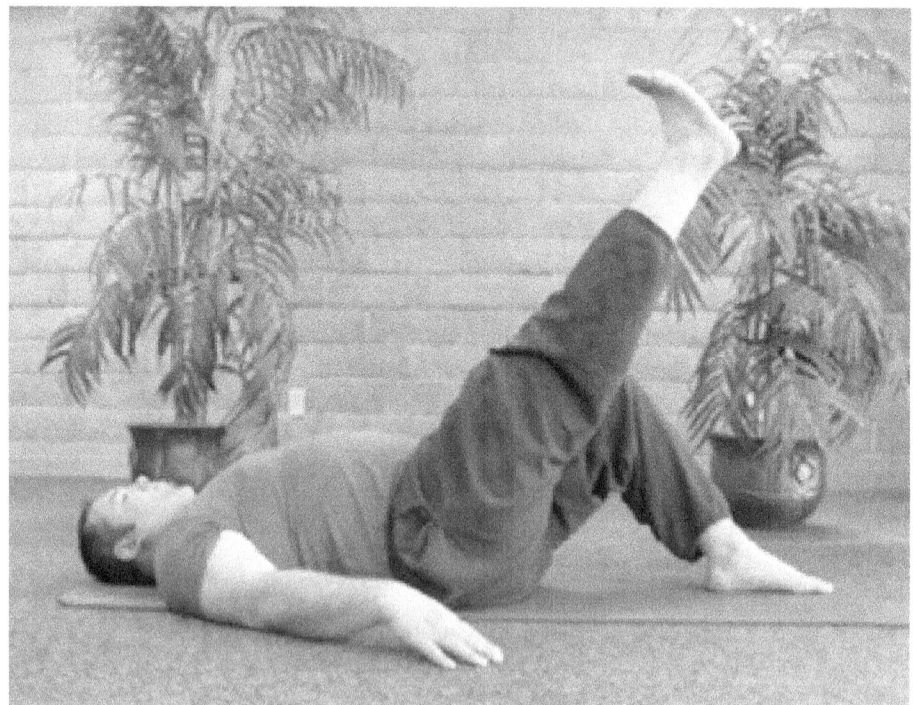

Extend the leg up and flex the foot.

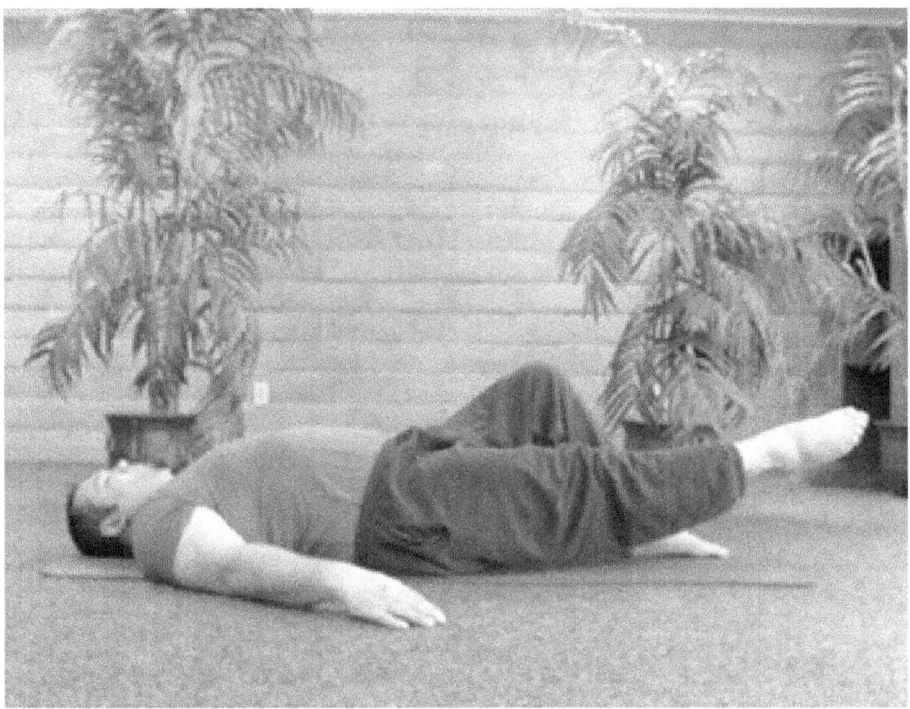

Lower the leg down with control.

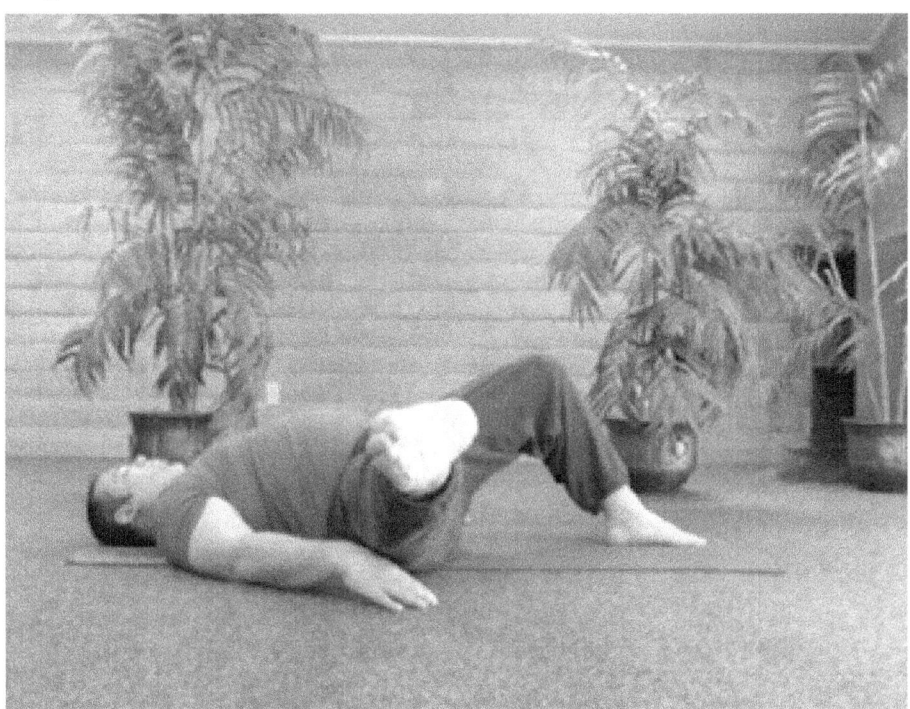

Point the toes. Keeping the strength in your core, rotate the leg pointing the toes outward, rotating from the hip. Extend the leg outward.

Bring the leg in using your inner thigh.

*This exercise has proved remarkable for removing inflammation in the knees. It's also helped rehabilitate those with weak musculature around the knee area.

SEALING YOUR PRACTICE

*It's very important that you don't skip this part. Please make time for yourself to heal by sealing your practice.

Relax on your back. You may put a small folded towel beneath your head, beneath your hips and the backs of your knees if you wish.

Let the arms rest out from the body with the palms turned up. Let the legs relax, as the feet fall outward.

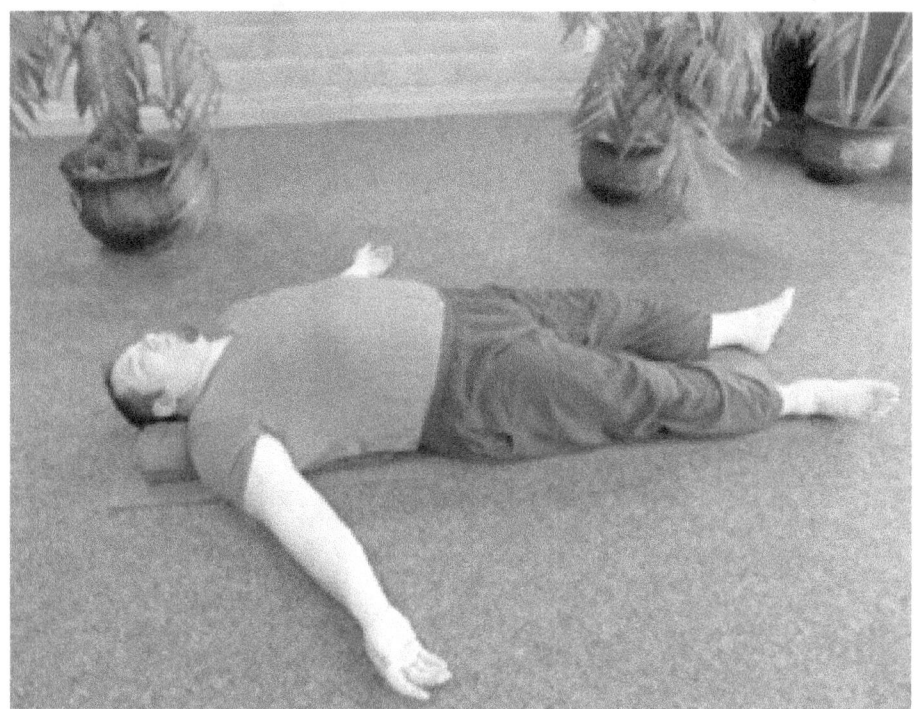

Release all tension. Breathe deep for several breaths and then let go completely. Unwind so much that you feel as if you are melting into the floor. Drift until your body becomes light, dissolving all worries and stress. Just let go.

This practice frees your nervous system of congested tension and sends signals to the muscles and brain to open and heal. There may be moments when you feel emotional in this state. Don't fight it. Let it come out, flowing from you until there is a great stillness within.

Stay in this practice for a minimum of three minutes.

When coming out, roll onto your left side and slowly come up. Sit tall in easy pose. Take two cleansing breaths and bring your palms together at the heart center. Welcome the peace of new life.

Please let this book be a guide into beginning your road to recovery. Keep passion in your heart and hope alive in miracles. The Technique is my gift after a long journey through debilitating chronic pain. Helping others through this work has given me great faith in the power of healing through the body and the human spirit.

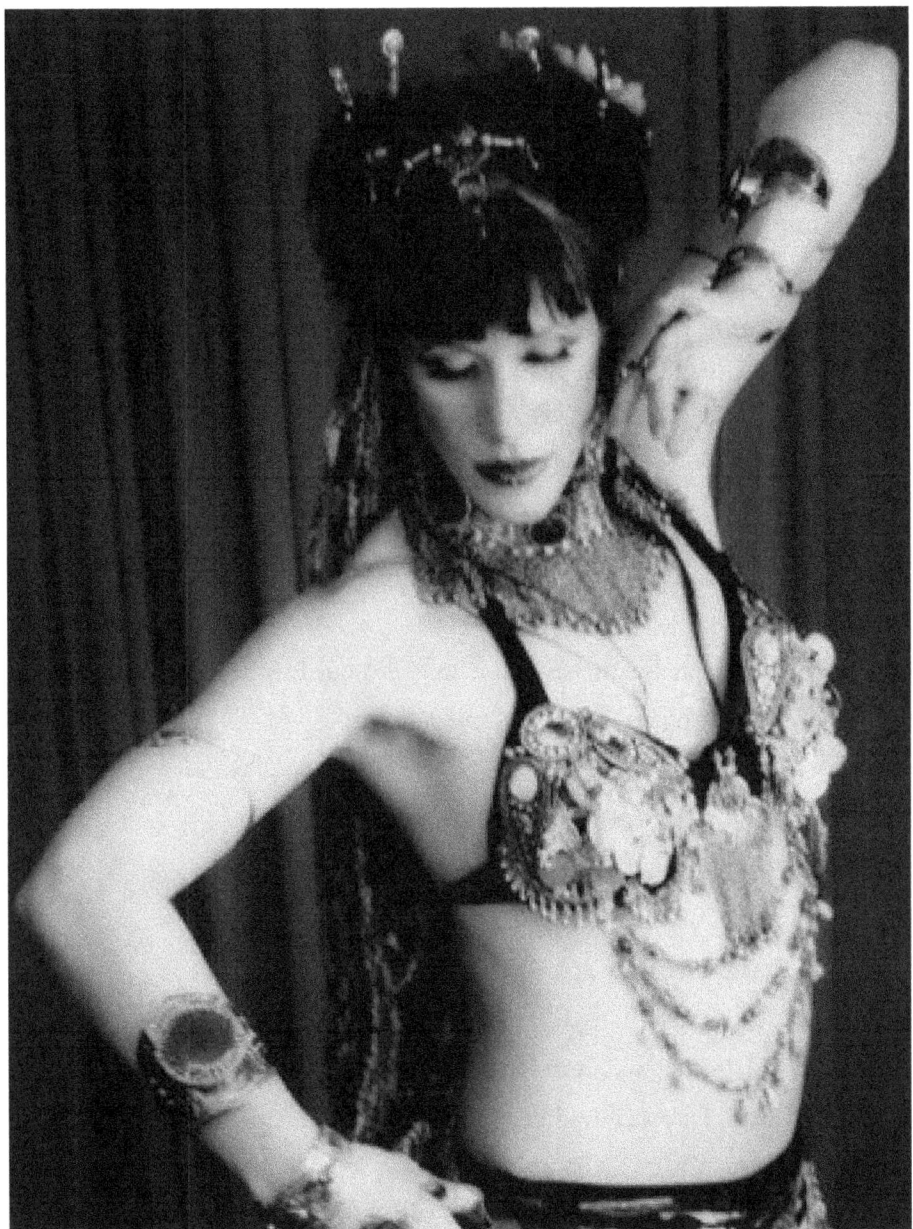

This book is dedicated to everyone with a passion to heal. It's not what happens to us in life but it's what we do with it that matters.

Blessings.

For more information about workshops and events please visit

www.juliet-cameron.com

Photo courtesy of Denise Marino

References/ Recommended Reading/ Documentaries

www.RemediesDirect.com

www.toothsoap.com

www.natural-health-information-centre.com

www.all-about-juicing.com

www.rawfoodlife.com

www.juicing-for-health.com

www.naturalcosmetics.com

www.globalhealingcenter.com

www.vibrancyuk.com

www.huffingtonpost.com

www.examiner.com

The Gerson Institute: www.gerson.org

Jay The Juice Man: www.jaykordich.com

Melvin Page D.D.S, H. Leon Abrams Jr.: 'Your Body is Your Best Doctor'

Dr. Weston A. Price: 'Nutrition and Physical Degeneration'

Dr. Lynn Tan: 'You Can Regain Youth and Health through Detoxification and Rejuvenation'

Publication 2003/ European Journal of Cancer Prevention

Dr. Christine Northrup: 'Women's Bodies, Women's Wisdom'

Dr. Herbert Shelton: 'Food Combining Made Easy'

The Journal of The American College of Toxicology

AJT Reports/ Studies on Sodium Lauryl Sulfate

Gerson Miracle/ 2004, Directed by: Steve Kroschel

Hungry for Change/ 2012, Directed by: James Colquhoun, Laurentine Ten Bosch

Fat, Sick and Nearly Dead/ 2010 Directed by: Joe Cross, Kurt Engfebr